THE ORAL HEALTH BIBLE

Michael P. Bonner, D.D.S., &
Earl L. Mindell, R.Ph., Ph.D.

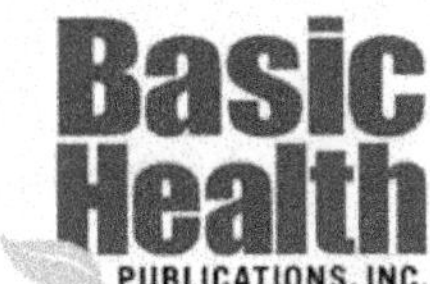

The information contained in this book is based upon the research and personal and professional experiences of the authors. It is not intended as a substitute for consulting with your physician or other healthcare provider. Any attempt to diagnose and treat an illness should be done under the direction of a healthcare professional.

The publisher does not advocate the use of any particular healthcare protocol but believes the information in this book should be available to the public. The publisher and authors are not responsible for any adverse effects or consequences resulting from the use of the suggestions, preparations, or procedures discussed in this book. Should the reader have any questions concerning the appropriateness of any procedures or preparation mentioned, the authors and the publisher strongly suggest consulting a professional healthcare advisor.

Basic Health Publications, Inc.
www.basichealthpub.com

Library of Congress Cataloging-in-Publication Data

Bonner, Michael P.

The oral health bible / Michael P. Bonner and Earl L. Mindell.
p. cm.
Includes bibliographical references and index.
ISBN 978-1-59120-050-5 (Pbk.)
ISBN 978-1-68162-814-1 (Hardcover)
1. Periodontal disease—Popular works. 2. Periodontal disease—Alternative treatment—Popular works. 3. Mouth—Diseases—Prevention—Popular works. 4. Dietary supplements—Popular works. I. Mindell, Earl. II. Title.

RK361.B66 2003
617.6'32—dc21
2003014249

Editor: Roberta W. Waddell
Typesetter: Gary A. Rosenberg
Cover design: Mike Stromberg

Contents

Foreword

Medical progress, viewed from outside the "Ivory Tower" would appear to be an unbroken series of new discoveries, zealously embraced from their inception by noble, unbiased, and selfless practitioners. Unfortunately, the history of medical science is really a history of new discoveries that languish for long intervals as their proponents toil for years shouting from the housetops to whomever will hear, until the world is finally ready to listen. Suddenly, an idea is recognized as valuable and essential. One example cited by the authors of this book is the development of the sterile technique. This concept of doctors washing their hands between examining patients, in order to prevent the spread of infection from one patient to the next, was first proposed by Ignaz Semmelweis in 1841. The results were spectacular. The practice dramatically reduced the rates of serious infection among mothers following deliveries in his maternity ward. Was Semmelweis declared a national hero? A medical genius? No. In fact, scandal and controversy erupted, and the practice of hand washing was immediately declared unnecessary and against official policy at his hospital. He was, in fact, summarily kicked out. Much later, as the germ theory of disease became accepted, the tide of change embraced hand washing, and we now take for granted the practice that Semmelweis began. He should have become a hero and his name a household word, but sadly, few outside medical circles know his name today.

Perhaps we like to think we are above such blind ignorance now, but looking back, it is apparent that the twentieth century was no different. Examples abound of great breakthroughs whose importance was initially obscured, and whose adoption was delayed by vain controversy, conformity, and obstinacy. That is, until the tide of change finally turned. The book you are holding now is a case in point; the tide of medical progress is turning again. As you will soon find out, the oral-systemic connection is a concept bolstered by years of research and reams of solid data that establishes, not just an ordinary connection, but a connection of incredible gravity and import. Simply put, people are dying for lack of knowledge of this ongoing health crisis. But, just as it was with Ignaz Semmelweis, simply presenting solid data is not enough. The data needs to be presented clearly, creatively, and tirelessly to the public and to enough physicians and dentists, to finally win the day. We can only hope and expect that the yeoman's work begun by Dr. Mike Bonner over these past several years—especially in writing this seminal book co-authored by none other than the nutritional authority Dr. Earl Mindell—is about to turn the tide in favor of change with respect to the oral-systemic paradigmatic model.

Dentists are fond of saying that physicians never actually examine a patient's mouth; rather, they look right past the mouth and into the throat, missing volumes of pertinent data that illuminate systemic health. Dentists, on the other hand, like to say that the mouth is a window revealing the health of the body in general. In fact, they were saying this long before the oral-systemic connection was made. Now, more than a platitude, it needs to become a clarion cry. Now, physicians need to learn to use this window on the body and act on the data revealed there. Dentists, on the other hand, need to learn they can and should have a profound impact on a patient's overall health, simply by enhancing oral health. What was formerly perceived as a window might more appropriately be called a doorway—to enhanced health, performance, and protection for all the body systems, but especially for the cardiovascular and immune systems.

The oral-systemic connection is about integration: the integrative paradigm. No longer just a buzz phrase, integrative medicine is beginning to fulfill its promise of recasting our view of the body and of health and healthcare, in general, into one about *connections and wholeness* rather than a minefield of artificially and dangerously disconnected parts. It seems obvious that the mouth is connected to the body, but we have not been treating it that way. We have had *mouth medicine* and *body medicine.* No wonder neither discipline fulfilled its true promise of solving the enigma of the oral-systemic connection. In this era of new, integrative medical concepts, such as mind/body medicine, the oral-systemic connection is right at home.

This book is also squarely astride another powerful movement in healthcare: the movement toward people taking responsibility for their own health, taking charge of their own bodies. This trend is sweeping away much of the chaff of healthcare, which accumulated when we gave away responsibility for our health to anyone but ourselves. By providing an action plan that allows us to take charge of our oral health, the authors empower us to have an impact on our systemic health. Will you be spared a myocardial infarction or a stroke because you read this book and took charge of your oral health? It is within the realm of possibility. Are you going to find out you have been approaching oral health in the wrong way? Yes, very probably so.

Speaking as a physician, I feel that a book about health isn't of much value if it doesn't lead me to modify something I do, whether that means adopting a new strategy or omitting an old one. If that is any measure of the importance of a book, let me just say: Get ready to change, because this book has made me take some U-turns in my own approach to oral health. In fact, in spite of my training, I find that, for the first time, I understand fundamental issues in oral health I knew little or nothing about, issues that my dentist apparently knows little about as well. Maybe I will be one of those spared a heart attack. I have thrown away my mouthwash, changed my toothpaste, and realized the limitations of flossing (which I thought was the holy grail of personal oral hygiene). Most important, I have had my suspicions that nutrition is paramount soundly confirmed. After reading this book, you will know your mouth, and you will never view it, or treat it, the same way again. There will be nothing abstract about the change that will occur in your own oral-systemic connection.

In spite of the serious topics addressed, this book is written the way health books ought to be: all terminology is well defined and explained, and, although oversimplification is avoided, there is a clarity that makes the book accessible. It is medical writing done right, and it is a pleasure to read. From volatile sulfur compounds and C-reactive protein to the anatomy of a sulcus, you will receive a painless education in oral health that will have you holding your own with the experts in no time. I chuckle to think how many of you who read this book will go back and educate your own dentists and physicians. Will your doctor remember you as the first patient who asked to have their CRP level checked when, many years from now, they are ordering them as routinely as they order cholesterol testing now?

Who would guess that the data would lead us to the knowledge that heart attacks, strokes, premature births, rheumatic diseases, and perhaps many more conditions would be so intimately linked to oral health and hygiene? The answer is that, just five years ago, very few people would have guessed this. But the authors of this volume knew then, and those of us fortunate enough to be reading this book will know very soon, that another health revolution has arrived. The oral-systemic connection is real, and we now have a pathway by which to transform health for many people who have been frustrated by chronic health problems that persist in spite of the state-of-the-art care they thought they were receiving. Now, thanks to Drs. Bonner and Mindell, we all have a new action plan on the road to peak health. Many thanks to the authors. I know your work is about to bear wonderful fruit by way of thousands of lives touched and changed—the greatest tribute any true healers can receive.

—Marcus L. Gitterle, M.D., B.C.E.M., A.B.A.A.M.
Diplomate, Board of Certification in Emergency Medicine
Diplomate, American Board of Anti-Aging Medicine
Wimberley, Texas

Preface

We are literally on the very leading edge of a health and wellness revolution in dentistry, and you'll soon see why in this book. As a dentist myself, I know that we *need* to be on the leading edge since dentists are supposed to be trained in diagnosing and treating dental diseases, especially the almost ubiquitous malady known as periodontal (gum) disease. Unfortunately, we have a really big problem because, first of all, gum disease is so prevalent that more people have it than don't, and second, because gum disease carries very serious health risks. Death certificates have probably never listed periodontal disease as the cause of death, but clear evidence has emerged implicating it as a major health risk and a cause of heart attacks and strokes, which do show up on death certificates.

What to do? Fortunately for all of us, there are safe, effective, and user-friendly answers to the gum-disease problem, and if we are successful at improving our oral health, our whole system should become healthier as well. Since when is oral health separate from the body it's attached to? It's my opinion that a major shift in how we view gum disease, and what we do about it, is seriously overdue. People *are* dying from the effects of gum disease, and unfortunately, the techniques and products commonly used by patients, in an honest attempt to be healthy, simply don't deliver the desired results in most instances.

With the growing awareness of gum disease's serious health consequences, dentists and patients alike are going to be looking for solutions in an attempt to get a better grip on this developing situation.

While all this is being sorted out in the dental profession, and I can assure you it will be, please pay close attention to what's in this book. It can help you take charge of your own oral health while we as a profession are establishing guidelines in standards of care. As an aside, I want you to know that I like and respect dentists. Dentistry is a tough profession, but the stakes are getting much higher with the almost daily revelations about gum disease and its serious consequences.

As an observer of the profession for more than twenty-eight years, I know change frequently comes slowly. However, what I have no appreciation for in my field is tolerating gum disease or the products, methods, or techniques that either do nothing, create additional disease, or simply make the existing gum disease worse. Products that carry scary warnings don't do so just for your reading pleasure.

I personally owe a large debt of gratitude to all the pioneers in health and wellness who have assisted me along the way, with an extra special dose going to Dr. Earl L. Mindell, who has patiently tolerated my well-meant suggestions over the last several years, while allowing me sufficient time to realize that he's a number of years ahead of me!

Additionally, many thanks go to Marcus Gitterle, M.D., for bringing C-reactive protein (CRP)—in the news almost daily now—to my attention four years ago, and for encouraging me to join the American Academy of Anti-Aging Medicine (A4M). It's been an interesting journey, and had they not opened the window for me, allowing me to look through and see the future of health and wellness, this book would not exist today. That being said, let's get on with it, as I expect you want to know how you can take control of your own oral health and systemic health. Oral health *is* systemic health.

The first purpose of this book is to assist you in better understanding just how serious periodontal (gum) disease is to your health. Although it is a disease that almost every adult in the United States has to some degree right now, very few realize that gum disease can have very serious systemic health consequences, including arteriosclerosis, diabetic complications, heart attacks, low-birth-weight babies, lung infections, strokes, and more. Gum disease isn't just bad breath, bleeding gums, and tooth loss anymore. It's far worse. As a dentist for more than twenty-eight years, I'm disturbed because new patients walking into my practice today have as much, or more, gum disease than was the case twenty-eight years ago. In this book, you will discover a number of reasons for this, and you may be appalled when you find out what's happening.

Right now we have a glaring dilemma in dentistry because, on the one hand, almost every adult walking around today has some form of periodontal disease, and on the other hand, we have a dental industry with a wide array of ADA-approved products containing ingredients that dozens of studies indicate can do more harm than good. A big example would be mouthwashes that government statistics indicate *cause* 36,000 cases of oral cancer a year, and kill approximately 500 people from alcohol ingestion. All this from mouthwashes that do nothing to improve oral health, yet the unknowing public trusts that these products will help them. Yet, there *are* health-enhancing alternative products available that will help, and this book will tell you what they are and where to find them.

Consider the oral health benefits attributed to daily brushing and flossing. The best brushers and flossers on the planet can still have gum disease because these tools do not effectively clean under the gums. You'll find out that there are devices to do this job handily that you've probably never heard of, and you'll learn where to get what you need. The brushing and flossing problem is similar to hosing down the roof to put out a fire that's in the basement.

Diagrams will show anatomically why brushing and flossing fall short of delivering the health benefits we expect from doing both activities on a daily basis. Keep doing both, of course, but realize they have their limitations.

The second purpose of this book is to look at the paradox involved in the potentially enormous benefit to your oral and systemic health that can be derived from the use of safe, effective nutritional supplements. The paradox lies in the fact that most, if not all, of the good information you need for robust gum and body health comes from sources outside dentistry. Most of the information I've used over the years has come from works written by people with Ph.D. or M.D. degrees, not D.D.S. or D.M.D. degrees. I don't understand why this is so, and there may be useful works written by dental health professionals that I am not aware of, but a recent search of every health, wellness, and nutrition-oriented book on Amazon.com revealed no titles available from dentists, and only a few available from dental authors on other dental subjects. I expect that will change in the near future, however, because we can't be casual about gum disease anymore. It is too serious a health challenge.

The information presented in this book is what I adhere to every day with my own patients, so it is benefiting them right now. While I have noted almost across-the-board health improvements, a recent example might serve as an illustration for health-improving possibilities. As you read this, please remember that, because I practice dentistry, not medicine, my recommendations were focused on my patient's gum disease.

Sarah—a middle-aged woman who was overweight, had high blood pressure, was tired and depressed, and also had moderate to severe periodontal disease, with pus and bleeding around several teeth—came to see me. Sarah said she was also experiencing abdominal pain in an area where surgery had been performed months before.

To prepare her for the required gum treatments by my dental hygienist three weeks hence, she was instructed to take a very complete all-natural supplement (120 balanced ingredients) daily, and to use a safe and effective organic toothpaste twice a day. Here I want to mention that the supplement she took was formulated by Dr. Earl L. Mindell, one of the original founders of the health and wellness revolution, and author of the best-selling book *The Vitamin Bible* (10 million copies sold to date). Sarah's success story will serve to illustrate why you might want to incorporate something similar into your own home-care program.

Three weeks later, when Sarah appeared for her first appointment with my dental hygienist, we saw a new person walking in. After just three weeks of brushing a couple of times a day with a toothpaste that's safe and effective, and taking two tablets of the supplement twice a day with major meals, an enthusiastic, smiling Sarah told the hygienist that her abdominal pain had gone away, she was no longer depressed, and she had enough energy to walk several miles a day. She had lost eleven pounds, her blood pressure was down, and, not surprisingly, her gum-tissue color and overall tissue tone was much healthier. All these positive health benefits occurred *before* any definitive dental treatment had begun. No dentist or hygienist had done anything more than examine Sarah and recommend a pretreatment program that would assist her in healing and make her treatment less hazardous. She had done all this herself.

Does this sound potentially worthwhile for you or someone you know? While it's impossible to guarantee similar results for anyone else, Sarah accomplished her substantial health improvements very quickly, using products that supported her in becoming healthier. And this example isn't unusual. The only unusual thing is that more people aren't taking advantage of what's already available.

Nutritional supplements, especially the top ten for oral health, are required to assist the body's immune system, as well as support the formation of collagen, the building block of connective tissue, cartilage, and bone. Gum tissue around the teeth is either totally intact, being the true effective barrier it is meant to be, or it is not, and if that is the case, the microorganisms are free to penetrate that barrier and circulate throughout the body. A boat floats, or it doesn't; there is no middle ground.

While we are blazing trails here in the oral health and wellness arena, the additional health benefits that I have frequently seen show me quite clearly that people can take a much more proactive role in their own health outcomes—safely and effectively. It will be a few more years before gum disease is recognized as the serious health issue it has been all along, but for now there's ample help that anyone can utilize to become healthier right now. That's what this book is about.

—Michael P. Bonner, D.D.S.
Member, American Dental Association
Member, Texas Dental Association
Member, Academy of General Dentistry
Member, American Academy of Anti-Aging Medicine

Acknowledgments

I offer my sincerest gratitude and humble thanks to the many dental patients who have trusted and accepted my health and wellness recommendations over the last several years. While it was never my intention to author a book based on my observations, your consistently positive results and enthusiasm for better health required that I pass this information on to others. I hope this effort honors your contribution.

Marcus Gitterle, M.D., has provided invaluable assistance and direction to my efforts over the last several years by sharing his medical perspective on systemic diseases, ostensibly of dental origin, and their potential amelioration through complementary methods. This section would be lengthy, indeed, if every important bit of information Dr. Gitterle has shared with me were enumerated here, so let me just say that your assistance, as well as your friendship, has not gone unnoticed. Thanks, Marcus.

Dr. Earl L. Mindell is in a league all his own. His efforts in educating the public on health and wellness issues with 300 radio and TV appearances a year, as well as 22 million books sold to date, means there is a public hungry for the information he provides. In the considerable number of conversations I've had with Dr. Mindell over the years, he has kindly allowed me to take as long as it took to figure things out on my own; most of the things I was concerned about, he'd thought of twenty or more years ahead of me, but I got it, finally. Thanks for everything you have done to help bring this book into existence. Your assistance has been incredible.

Beginning when this book was just an idea, and continuing throughout, Linda Chaé has been infinitely resourceful in finding nutritional research material for my consideration. Her generosity is amazing. Additionally, Linda was one of the first people to identify the myriad of harmful ingredients that are almost universally included in most of the personal-care items people use every day (she terms these ingredients "the untouchables"). She also testified before the United States Congress in late 2001 concerning the harmful effects that these untouchables have upon their user's health. Linda has not only identified a very serious problem, but she is also doing something about it. She has pioneered the development of safe, effective products for our personal use and is, in fact, the developer of the oral health products that work so well for my patients. Bravo, Linda.

Many thanks go to the following people for their considerable help in this effort: M. F. Black, my mother, who early on instilled in me a love for reading and language; Rosemary Kitten for her considerable patience on this project; Michelle Olson, my very capable dental assistant; Dr. Scott Barton, D.D.S., for his support. Drs. Perry Marcel and Jose M. Gonzalez are due thanks as well, since they are both busy practicing dentists whose in-office health and wellness activities have mirrored mine, with similar results. Additionally, K. C. and Petey, my two loyal cats, although seldom awake, were ever present during this project.

Finally, I graciously acknowledge Roberta (Bobby) Waddell, who patiently and expertly edited this book. Her support, enthusiasm, and insight into the topics covered, including a broad understanding of nutrition, have all been woven into creating the message I wanted the reader to get, and I feel she has done a most commendable job. Thanks, Bobby!

Introduction

A check for periodontal (gum) disease would reveal that at least nine out of ten adults have some evidence of gum disease at this time, and it would be safe to say that very few of them know they have it (it's generally painless until it's too late). Gum disease isn't just the major cause of tooth loss and bad breath anymore. Even though both of these conditions are serious enough by themselves, periodontal disease is a far more serious health condition than either bad breath or tooth loss because it is very closely associated with several systemic health conditions, including arteriosclerosis, heart attacks, lung disease, premature births, rheumatoid arthritis, strokes, and more. In fact, the connection between periodontal disease and these severe systemic conditions has been confirmed by studies reported in the dental media. There is a common link in all this and it is largely avoidable, but only if the person with the gum disease knows what to do.

The fact is, if a person decided today to try and take control of, or even reverse, their gum disease by making changes in their home-care efforts, the odds are nearly 100 percent that they would be unsuccessful, and that they would likely damage their health further by using products purportedly formulated to combat gum disease that are actually harmful—products such as commonly available mouthwashes and toothpastes.

Anyone who has ever eaten hot peppers or other spicy foods has observed the burning sensation in their mouth, and how long this sensation lingers while the substances get absorbed. I know I have, and nothing would reduce the pain. The burn just had to wear itself out because, painful or not, oral soft tissues are great at absorbing whatever comes in contact with them. It is very unfortunate that consumers unknowingly use oral health products every day that most likely contain ingredients known to cause health problems, not improve them, because these harmful products also get absorbed into the soft mouth tissues. Does anyone honestly believe that antifreeze (propylene glycol), formaldehyde, sodium lauryl (and laureth) sulfate, sodium hydroxide, and even triclosan, an EPA-registered pesticide similar in chemical structure to dioxin, have any health-enhancing benefits when they are absorbed into the soft oral tissues on their way to being stored in the body? I doubt it, but, unfortunately, two or more of these ingredients are in most toothpastes you are likely to be using right now.

Mouthwash that is up to 60-proof alcohol offers no worthwhile benefits either, considering the risks, such as oral cancer (36,000 cases a year) or alcohol-ingestion deaths (500 cases a year). It can even dissolve cosmetic dental materials. And, as if the alcohol content isn't bad enough, mouthwash formulators include known carcinogens, such as phenol, as well as potentially harmful coloring agents, to make these dangerous rinses red, blue, yellow, green, and so on. What I'm saying is, most people trust and use products that have the potential to hurt them rather than help them.

It gets worse. Part of an effective home-care program is to clean the area under the gums (the sulcus) on a regular basis, preferably every day. But how can a toothbrush clean under the gum margin? (By the way, only *soft* or *ultra-soft* brushes should ever be used in the mouth. Medium and hard brushes are great for cleaning small motor parts and boots, not teeth.) While effective toothbrushing is an essential daily oral health activity, it does have its limitations. How about floss? Flossing is another essential daily oral health activity that delivers obvious benefits, especially if done properly every day, but can it really clean under the gums? It won't clean very well, and definitely *not* below the gum margin edges, where the most serious problems occur. Floss will go no lower than the gum tissue on the cheek and the tongue sides of the tooth will let it; and unfortunately, it simply can't clean the sulcus, the space between each tooth and the gum tissue surrounding it that harbors microorganisms, dead gum-tissue cells, and food debris—not a pretty situation. There are, however, devices that can do this important job handily, and they are easy to use.

Another area that is presently underappreciated in clinical dentistry, and therefore generally missing as an integral, recommended part of any effective oral health program, is the potentially exceptional health benefit provided by a wide array of totally safe and very effective nutritional supplements. With heart attacks, cancer, and strokes listed as the top three causes of death in this country in 2001 (prescription drugs come in at number four, with 265,000 deaths), it would clearly be a good idea to take advantage of supplements that not only help to make the gums healthier, but also contribute to heart health, increased energy, weight loss (if needed), reduced cancer risk, and lower cholesterol—all with total safety and without the possibility of drug reactions. This book will discuss the many supplements that can work wonders at safely alleviating these and other conditions.

Please be aware that all recommendations for nutritional supplements come from exceedingly reputable sources, including books such as Dr. Earl Mindell's *Vitamin Bible for the 21st Century* and the *PDR for Nutritional Supplements,* both of which could serve as valuable resources for you in taking better control of your health. Additionally, Dr. Earl Mindell provided much of the information in Chapter 8, including the top ten nutrients for a healthy mouth. I encourage you to be open-minded enough to consider any of the recommendations that may be appropriate to your situation, and judge for yourself whether there is a benefit. At the same time, though, I encourage you to be skeptical and do your own "due diligence" when it comes to your health. I will make quite a number of very specific recommendations for products and devices, and where there is more than one source, or no noticeable difference between products, I will leave it to you to choose. High-quality products are generally more expensive than their lower-priced competitors, and while additional monthly expenses for better health can put a strain on some patients' budgets, I have occasionally pointed out to my patients that gum surgery, angioplasty, even funerals don't come cheap either.

In addition, it would be helpful to have information on specific markers—such as your cholesterol (HDL and LDL) levels, C-reactive protein level (measured by a high-sensitivity CRP test), weight, blood pressure, and blood-sugar level—before you begin a program that could very well improve these numbers over time.

I also recommend a medical checkup as part of a prevention-oriented home-care program, and I promise you that your physician *will* be interested in seeing you get healthier. In addition, there are oral health products that can have a profoundly beneficial effect on joint health and comfort, so, once again, while our goal is to improve oral health, there are systemic benefits that go along with it. Take the examples of methylsulfonylmethane (MSM) and Zincosamine (a safe, nonprescription Cox-II inhibitor—Vioxx and Celebrex are the two prescription Cox-II inhibitors you may have seen advertised on TV): peer-reviewed studies substantiate their anti-inflammatory activity and their lack of toxicity or harmful side effects.

I have written this book to make it possible for you to improve your oral and systemic health in ways you may not have thought possible. If you have any doubts, consider that many of my patients follow some or all of the recommendations in this book every day, and they are all measurably healthier because of it. I hope to demystify periodontal disease and simplify how you can protect yourself from it. As the book's title implies, effective oral health products, devices, and techniques do offer a pathway to optimal health. If you take advantage of the information presented here, you will be rewarded with measurably positive results.

It is unfortunate that, at the present time, health and wellness activities in standard dentistry tend only toward the traditional, and give only traditional results. I believe that dentists need to get far more involved in their patients' health challenges than they currently do, because there is so much we can safely help them accomplish, knowing that the health of the mouth mirrors the health of the whole body.

My recommendations, however, are not intended as substitutes for traditional methods of oral healthcare. You will still need to partner with your dentist, and I encourage you to be open with her or him because, if you are doing the best you can at home with the recommendations from this book, it is practically a guarantee that your dentist or hygienist will notice. Healthy mouths are rare enough that they *will* notice the difference in you, but you'll notice it first. Someone once said, "If you keep doing what you've been doing, you'll keep getting what you've been getting," so I hope you agree with me that it's time for a whole new way of looking at, and dealing with, this ever present infection known as periodontal disease.

As the famous Mayo brothers said in 1910, almost one hundred years ago: *A person with a healthy mouth will live ten years longer.* We're just now learning why that statement rings true.

1

The Bad News about Gum Disease—It's Not Just Bad Breath, Cavities, and Loose Teeth

Periodontal disease has serious health consequences that go well beyond cavities, tooth loss, and halitosis (bad breath). Although approximately 90 percent of the public probably has some form of gum disease that can be easily detected by a dental health professional, those who bother to get checked for it are, in general, primarily concerned about keeping their teeth by having regular cleanings, getting any cavities filled before the tooth aches, and perhaps freshening their breath, or seeing about getting their teeth whitened. These are valid concerns, of course, but evidence suggesting that healthy gums are *required* in order to avoid other more serious health consequences continues to build. Current research has clearly shown that periodontal disease is a known factor for increased risk of heart attacks and strokes, in addition to being a cause of nearly one in five preterm births and a factor in rheumatoid arthritis. This list will get longer as it becomes increasingly apparent that a circulatory system swimming in microorganisms, which would be better confined to the mouth, is being subjected to a life-threatening assault. The bugs are winning at the present time, but we need to be winning, not the microorganisms. The focus of this book is to tip the balance in our favor.

While most researchers currently in the periodontal-systemic disease arena do not come right out and say that gum disease is a *definite* cause of a number of serious health problems, some medical doctors have helped people by writing books on how to do something about the horrific health consequences of a deep-seated, systemic infection.

These books have included complete chapters on the periodontal-systemic disease connection, along with very helpful, safe, and effective advice to follow to become healthier. It does seem paradoxical that physicians, not dentists, are the front-runners, by years, in providing the information the public needs to combat a very serious disease, but I'm just grateful that somebody is paying attention.

While I am all for more research and continued study in the role of periodontal disease and its systemic effects, studies on dental caries and periodontal disease have already consumed huge amounts of research money and time for decades; yet the public *still* has billions of unfilled cavities ripe with decay, and nine out of ten adults are known to have some evidence of gum disease. It is now time for the dental researchers to do something about making people a lot healthier. I'd like for them to look at and publicize methods, products, or devices that actually address the periodontal-systemic disease situation and take the lead in helping us with our problem. They can start by evaluating safe, effective oral health products (toothpastes and mouthwashes), hydromagnetic irrigators, and several classes of nutritional supplements, and then disseminate this information to those who may not be reading this book.

Safe, effective methods do exist and, interestingly, some of the nutritional elements necessary for better health have been around since the late 1920s (flavonoids, vitamin C), while other important nutrients have been working wonders for at least twenty-five years (CoQ_{10} and the proanthocyanidins). Hydromagnetics has been around for decades as well, so it is time to put all this and more to work.

The first and foremost way to get gum disease under better control is to rivet the public's attention on the fact that bleeding gums, loose teeth, and pus are definitely *not* okay. Healthy gums are meant to provide a barrier, keeping the approximately 400 types of microorganisms normally found in the mouth *in* the mouth and *not* circulating throughout the body, creating inflammatory mischief wherever the body is susceptible, including such places as the arterial wall where plaques form. Please be aware that just one gram of plaque can contain trillions of microorganisms, and the role of healthy gum tissue is to keep these out of the body.

Except for choosing our parents, we can control most of the factors that cause gum disease, but one fact is certain: either the gum tissue is an intact, complete barrier, or it is not. Any opening in the gum-tissue barrier allows microorganisms to enter the circulatory system, so the goal of any periodontal health program should be to regain and maintain a true soft-tissue barrier around the teeth. For this to happen, however, there has to be a dramatic shift in how gum disease is perceived and controlled.

An evaluation of the gum tissue itself would be a logical place to start. The skin barrier covering our bodies is a type of epithelium called stratified squamous. The cell shapes look like irregularly formed pancakes, and are derived from a basal layer of living tissue that produces the skin cells we see as skin; it also supplies the blood flow and elasticity of skin, allowing movement. The skin cells produced at the basal layer, no longer living by the time they reach the surface, are what we see as skin. These slough off continuously as new cells are generated below, from the basal layer. If our skin barrier is intact, with no openings due to cuts, scrapes, blisters, or other breaches of the barrier, we are safely protected inside the barrier (the skin)—even with potentially infectious microorganisms on the skin. Gum tissue is also this same stratified squamous epithelium, and except for a lack of hair follicles and being almost continuously moist, it is essentially similar to the tissue that's found on the back of our hands, and its function is also the same—to serve as a barrier to microorganisms.

A person with moderate to severe gum disease has inflamed and infected tissue wrapped around their teeth, with enough collective surface area to approximate the surface area you would see on the back of your hand, about nine to twelve square inches. Under the gums, there are up to 400 types of microorganisms, numbering in the trillions, all swimming, living, and dying in this necrotic stew around the teeth, creating major inflammation and odor. While we can't see this infected tissue around the teeth, it is there nonetheless. This fact helps bring to light how serious this hidden problem really is.

To get a sense of this, imagine that the entire back of your hand is wet, with redness, swelling, odor, and 400 types of microorganisms on it. Would this skin be raw? Would it be tender, and bleed when scratched? Wouldn't anyone with this problem understand intuitively that they were ill and do whatever it takes to get healthy once more, or would they continue to ignore the problem? If most people could see what is really going on, they would take gum disease far more seriously.

Two more questions are in order here. First, would a well-nourished person using supernutrients have this problem? Second, do you believe that pouring alcohol-based mouthwash (40–60 proof—60 proof equals 30 percent alcohol) on your infected hand would be a good idea?

I hope this explanation has proved helpful in visualizing how serious the problem of gum disease really is. We must begin to take it seriously.

Unfortunately, the skin cells that are continuously sloughing off under the gums provide a food source for the microorganisms living in the same space. As these cells decompose under the gums, they produce odors known as volatile sulfur compounds (VSCs). This toxic stew of VSC gases under the gums consists primarily of methyl mercaptan (sewer gas odor) and hydrogen sulfide (rotten egg odor). More unfortunate perhaps than the social problem of bad breath is the fact that both gases have been shown to activate protein-dissolving (proteolytic) enzymes that work to destroy the barrier.[1] In other words, *odors under the gums* can initiate periodontal disease by eroding the barrier. Although there is considerable help available in combating this situation, and you will read about it in this book, you should be aware that current home-care techniques and recommendations do not effectively deal with it. As vital to your daily routine as brushing and flossing are, they cannot clean under the gums where the stew is, nor can they neutralize VSC *or* increase gum-tissue resistance to the proteolytic enzymes.

One of the key problems with periodontal-systemic disease is overcoming the public's dangerously blasé attitude toward it. Very few people seem concerned, initially, when I gently check their gums with a probe and find there is bleeding. While dentists and hygienists are trained to assess whether the bleeding is delayed or immediate, to note how many areas bleed, to determine and record the depth of the pockets, and to note the presence or absence of suppuration (pus), the profession and the public alike still view oral disease as if it were somehow removed from the rest of the body. It is not. A person with bleeding gum tissue, bone loss, and pus around even one tooth is at risk of more than just a bill for dental services; that person is systemically ill. Veterinarians have been tuned in to the health consequences of gum disease in animals for years. The American Veterinary Medical Association recently reported that tartar and gingivitis, which are both involved in gum disease and are present in both animals and humans, were the *first* and *second* most serious pet health problems.[2] So, if gum diseases and their consequences are rated at the very top of the list of most serious health problems in animals, perhaps medicine and dentistry should follow suit and rate them the same for humans. If gum disease were painful, it might get more attention, but unfortunately it is not. It is generally silent and painless until it is well advanced, which is a good reason to have your mouth regularly checked for signs of disease by a competent dentist. (In the future, a blood test that looks at circulating inflammatory components, such as C-reactive protein, will be a routine part of a thorough dental health examination, as it is now for many of my patients.)

What's so bad about gum disease? Hundreds of studies have looked at different aspects of the gum disease–systemic disease connection, and have found it can be a causative factor in a heart attack or stroke, two of the top three causes of death. Studies have shown that gum disease can increase the risk of a heart attack by 200 to 400 percent, as well as double the risk of a stroke. Infant mortality is affected by gum disease, and there are ongoing studies showing that, with as few as two diseased sites, mothers can experience premature birth or low-birth-weight babies. Other studies have shown that gum disease can make arteriosclerosis and diabetes worse, and can even contribute to lung disease caused by breathing in (aspirating) pneumonia-causing organisms.

Gum disease is not something you want to have, principally because gum-disease inflammation creates circulating substances called proinflammatory cytokines, which the liver modifies into C-reactive protein (CRP), a very hazardous entity. CRP causes clotting and, depending on where the clot occurs, can cause a heart attack, a stroke, a deep vein thrombosis in a leg, or even a pulmonary embolus. Since CRP is inflammation-induced, any source of inflammation, such as arthritis, can increase CRP levels. And since gum disease is a major producer of inflammation throughout the body, and therefore a major contributor to increased CRP levels in the majority of people, we need to focus our attention on total body inflammation in order to reduce those levels.

The medical profession is currently coming to the conclusion that high CRP levels are as serious a threat to health as high cholesterol (an acknowledged cause of heart attacks and strokes), and doctors are beginning to screen for this blood element as part of regular health checkups. CRP has even made it into *Readers' Digest* (April 2002, p.113), in a short piece stating that CRP testing "may be getting ready for prime time" because it is a highly predictive marker for signs of inflammation. Since CRP is produced in the liver, and this production is triggered by inflammation anywhere in the body, a high CRP reading would be the result of that person's total cumulative inflammation. Someone with severe arthritis, prostate inflammation, and healthy gums could have a high CRP reading, just as someone with severe periodontal disease and no arthritis or other inflammatory problems could. Regardless of the source, it all adds up, and high CRP levels are dangerous no matter what disease caused them. But, since gum disease is an inflammation-inducing condition that more people have than don't, it has to be considered a primary culprit in many disease processes, including that of elevated CRP levels.

CRP levels are usually measured in milligrams per liter (mg/L) and, as reported in an article in the *San Antonio Express-News,*[3] CRP levels of less than 1 mg/L indicate a low risk for heart disease, and readings between 1 and 3 mg/L represent an average risk. CRP levels higher than 3 mg/L indicate high risk, and people with CRP levels greater than 3 mg/L are at least twice as likely to develop cardiovascular disease as those in the low-risk group.

The danger of gum disease to overall health is dose related, which means the worse the gum disease, the greater the risk. Severe inflammation elsewhere in the body is serious as well. (Please remember this connection since oral health recommendations presented later in this book have been shown not only to improve oral health, but also to offer relief from a number of other health problems, including arthritis.)

As reported in the Spring 2002 issue of *The Mission* (published by the University of Texas Health Science Center at San Antonio), it has been estimated that up to 400 specific types of microorganisms are commonly indigenous to the mouth, so with gum disease there is the distinct likelihood that several types of these potentially hazardous microorganisms are circulating throughout the entire body, wherever the blood flow takes them. In a study reported in the October 2000 issue of *Compendium,* a postmortem examination of blood clots taken from arteries in the neck showed several types of disease-causing bacteria in the clots of 72 percent of the recently deceased test subjects (fifty clots from the carotid arteries were evaluated during these autopsies).

When the inflammation-induced nature of CRP is considered, other life-threatening aspects should be taken into account, so please read the following carefully. When a person with moderate to severe periodontal disease and elevated CRP levels undergoes a deep cleaning (scaling and root planing), what happens to the CRP levels as the dentist or hygienist tears the diseased tissues in their normal efforts to treat gum disease? (I can tell you from experience that diseased gum tissues are quite fragile and easily torn.) There are a number of unexpected results that may occur in anyone undergoing periodontal procedures, perhaps even ones as innocuous as everyday scaling and root planing. Studies have shown that periodontal cleaning procedures alone can elevate the person's baseline CRP readings by 300 percent. This rise can be truly life-threatening for anyone who has advanced gum disease, since acute infection can elevate CRP levels to 500 to 1,000 times already high normal limits. If a CRP reading of 3 mg/L is considered high risk for a cardiovascular event, imagine how much more hazardous it would be to have CRP levels in the 1,500–3,000 mg/L range. It seems logical that scraping deep under the gums in infected, inflamed tissues would cause CRP levels to skyrocket even more.

Even extraordinarily high risk levels can be prevented or controlled by a wide variety of inflammation-reducing substances. Yet very few people ever receive pretreatment protection from their dentists unless they have a known heart problem, such as mitral valve prolapse, valvular damage from rheumatic fever, or some other condition, such as hip joint replacement, requiring pretreatment antibiotic coverage.

While critically important for those needing it, antibiotic coverage is not the same as anti-inflammatory coverage, which is a basically unknown procedure. With antibiotics, there is protection against the oral microorganisms that generally accompany professional oral hygiene procedures, but the increase of inflammation-induced CRP in almost everyone is ignored. CRP levels will soar unless steps are taken to reduce or eliminate this tangible risk. So preparing yourself by taking anti-inflammatory supplements well before undergoing periodontal procedures is a good and necessary step toward keeping the CRP levels under control. Better safe than sorry, so if your dentist doesn't recommend it, do it yourself. Such pretreatment will help you heal faster, and more comfortably, with less swelling and bruising. Any number of substances can offer protection from inflammation-induced CRP elevation, but the physicians I have consulted all agree on taking a specific dosage of chewable vitamin C just prior to gum treatments.

Gum disease treatment actually increases inflammation *dramatically,* by elevating proinflammatory cytokines, which, in turn, elevate CRP production in the liver. When I have brought this risk factor to the attention of my patients over the last several years, many of them have informed me that one or more of their friends or relatives have suffered either a stroke or a heart attack anywhere from twenty-four hours to two weeks after having periodontal procedures done. In one four-month period alone, three of my patients reported five deaths such as this in their own families. While my observations do not constitute a scientific study, anecdotal incidents such as these are undoubtedly occurring elsewhere. It is clear to me that the dental patients of the world could use some help right now; I believe the scientific community would do well to study the incidence of mortality and morbidity associated with periodontal procedures, and not only increase awareness of the problem but also help design regimens to reduce the risk.

In summary, while most dental scientists won't come right out and say that gum disease is a definite cause of heart attacks and strokes, they do acknowledge an apparent connection, mainly because the current dental literature is edging closer to recognizing the intimate connection between gum disease and diabetes, heart attacks, low-birth-weight babies, rheumatoid arthritis, and strokes.

If history is any indication of what the future may bring, the dental profession is in for a big change. In the mid- and late-nineteenth century, surgeons did not have the concept of germs or bacteria and their direct role in causing infection, nor did they have any concept of sterilization and disinfection, so they did not bother to sterilize surgical instruments and surgical dressings, or practice scrupulous hand-washing techniques. Louis Pasteur and his discovery of the importance of animalcules, now known as bacteria, helped to usher in better hygiene as well as an understanding of the infectious disease-causing processes. But even after Pasteur's discovery, surgeons who were noted for being notably fastidious in matters of cleanliness were still ridiculed because surgical-sterility concepts took a while to catch on.

Before Pasteur, Ignaz Semmelweis accomplished his dramatic reduction of childbirth fever (which usually resulted in the death of the mother) by merely washing the bed linens and other items in germ-killing carbolic acid, instead of using the same linens and instruments over and over, on patient after patient. Incredibly enough, even with his rate of childbirth fever dropping consistently—90 percent or more compared to his physician peers (Semmelweis: one death; colleagues: ten deaths)—he was ostracized for years before his methods and concepts became common practice. What kind of defense can there be for a situation in which ten of their patients die for every one death of the individual they are ridiculing? Before looking askance at these skeptics, however, just be aware that our present-day blinders are every bit as good as they were back then, and personal points of view still tend to be held as totally infallible, to the general exclusion of any other possible point of view—until they are proven incorrect, which then necessitates a shift in how we look at things.

My modest hope is that this book will get people and the dental profession alike to look at periodontal health and systemic health in the new ways I am proposing. They'll appreciate having done so, I believe, when they see the overwhelming evidence supporting the safety and effectiveness of it. Gum disease is an epidemic right now, so it can't get much worse, and taking a look at other possibilities only requires an open mind.

An apt example of how views change radically can be demonstrated by the concept of laudable pus. There was a time when pus welling out of a surgical incision was thought to be a good (laudable) sign that the body was healing, but of course it was just the opposite. Today, we consider this concept outrageous, but once it was the norm. Similarly, although no responsible dental health professional would ever tell a patient that gum disease is actually good for them, we still have a long way to go before the profession accepts the many changes required to make people dramatically healthier than they are now. Dental health is intimately connected to systemic health, so change is hopefully on the way for both the profession and the people it treats.

The following chapters will help you understand how the changes you make will result in a positive, measurable difference in not just your oral health but also the health of your body overall.

2

"What Do You Mean I've Got Gum Disease? My Gums Always Bleed"

So many patients have said these words to me over the years that if I could get all of them to say it together simultaneously, I would have a chorus, also singing "they wouldn't bleed if you didn't poke them." While bleeding gums are considered normal, since it's so common for people to have gum disease, bleeding gums are also a sign of a potentially serious systemic disease. They are a clear indication that the barrier intended to keep microorganisms in the mouth and out of the circulatory system isn't properly performing its important role. Gum disease is not a healthful condition. My patients, whom I love and respect, may not intend to encourage periodontal disease, but they *are* doing so.

My deep concern lies in the fact that people with gum disease are, in fact, potentially seriously ill and do not even realize they have a problem, or if they do, think it's of no more consequence than a cold. The challenge for me is that this country is not up in arms over gum disease, because it is a disease so insidious, so painless, so seemingly benign—yet so dangerous—that it is allowed to affect perhaps 90 percent of the adult population, while we continue to pour oral health products containing antifreeze and alcohol on diseased gums. Heart disease alone kills the equivalent of six fully loaded 747 jumbo jets every day, about 2,190 jumbos a year, with deaths approaching 800,000 people. I say we've got to do a lot better than we do at present to address this dismal situation. And we can. If gum disease were as painful as a continuous bee sting or a burn, perhaps the hundred million or so Americans who have moderate to advanced gum disease would be ringing their physicians' and dentists' phones off the hook. This type of pain would serve to alert people to the fact that they did, in fact, have some sort of problem as well as motivate them to do something about it. Nothing of this sort will happen, of course, because gum disease is, as I said, usually painless, and bleeding gums aren't given much thought.

Since you are reading this book, I may be preaching to the converted, but we in the dental profession, and the population we treat, *must* take periodontal disease much more seriously. Not to do so bodes ill for making any progress in ameliorating the ravages of this ubiquitous, insidious disease.

How Do We Know If We've Got Gum Disease?

Periodontal disease literally means disease that is "located around a tooth"[1] and is generally meant to refer either to infections around the teeth, such as gingivitis, an early stage of periodontal disease, or to more deep-seated infections around the teeth resulting in pockets and the loss of tooth-supporting bone, known variously as early, moderate, or advanced periodontitis. Exact gradations of the disease range from simple, easily cured conditions requiring little professional therapy to exceedingly complex ones requiring therapy from a periodontist (a gum specialist). End-stage periodontal disease results in extraction, the only therapy possible, and thus the loss of the tooth. While the traditional perspective is a tooth-by-tooth, oral-centric focus, my perspective is that we should be thinking about early, moderate, and advanced *systemic* disease that shows up first in the mouth.

There can be many causes of periodontal disease, and someone can have several factors working against them at any given time. One of the biggest factors in determining whether or not you have gum disease is how well you can control plaque by exercising whatever oral hygiene efforts you customarily perform.

Plaque, the sticky stuff that coats the teeth above and below the gums, is a major factor in the development and perpetuation of gum disease. Since up to 400 types of microorganisms are living, dying, rotting, stinking, and producing a whole host of destructive enzymes under the gums, and therefore next to the teeth, plaque is very high on the list of periodontal disease causes. One gram of biofilm from any source, whether above or below the gum margins, or even from the top of the tongue, can contain as many as 100–200 trillion organisms (a heavy load for any mouth); therefore, safe, effective methods of controlling these organisms on a daily basis are critical to maintaining oral health.

Although poor oral hygiene and plaque control is frequently the primary cause of gum problems, there are also other factors that contribute to periodontal disease (even an immaculately clean mouth can be diseased). They include:

- Nutritional deficiencies (98 percent of the population fits into this category because, as a nation, we are overfed and undernourished);
- A diet high in sugar, white flour, and other refined carbohydrates (these foods depress the immune system);
- Diabetes (decreased resistance to infection, poor circulation);
- Alcohol (dehydration, poor diet, topical effect of alcohol on gums, vitamin depletion);
- Stress (compromised immune system);
- Bruxism (grinding) and malocclusion (bad bite);
- Volatile sulfur compounds (derived from decomposing food debris—VSC breaks down protein, decomposing microorganisms, desquamated cellular debris under the gums);
- Smoking, chewing, dipping, or using tobacco in any form (tobacco has many ill effects on oral soft tissues, including oral cancer and periodontal disease);
- Drug reactions, especially to the birth control pill and steroids (mouth-drying effects, reduced immune-system competency);
- Hereditary factors (not commonly seen, but in some, its influence shows up early and can quickly result in major bone loss and loss of teeth);
- Poorly fitting dental appliances (too much stress on remaining teeth), bad margins, or over- or undercontoured restorations or crowns;
- Food impaction between teeth (causing bone loss, chronic inflammation, localized pressure);

- Habits, such as chronic nail biting, improper use of toothpicks, and overzealous brushing or flossing;
- Foreign-body reaction (bone loss can occur rapidly when foreign material is lodged under the gums—popcorn hulls, tomato seeds, or toothpick remnants can all cause mischief in just days or weeks);
- Chronic immune diseases or HIV/AIDS infection;
- Inflammation, the chief culprit in most periodontal disease-systemic disease connections.

Robert Genco, D.D.S., Ph.D., editor-in-chief of the *Journal of Periodontology,* says, "It seems clear that gum disease, far from being just an oral health problem, actually represents a significant health risk to millions of people." Dr. Genco further states, "Periodontal disease is characterized by *inflammation* and bacterial infection of the gums surrounding the teeth. The bacteria that are associated with periodontal disease can travel in the bloodstream to other parts of the body, and that puts health at risk." Additionally, Dr. Genco says, "People think of gum disease in terms of their teeth, but they don't think about the fact that gum disease is a *serious infection* that can release bacteria into the bloodstream. The end result could mean additional health risks for people whose health is already affected by other diseases—or lead to serious complications like heart disease."[2]

While the list of factors playing a role in periodontal disease is extensive, and despite the dire (and correct) warnings of Dr. Genco, the good news is that most of these factors (genetics excepted) are under our control. Even though we still have no say in picking our parents, all is not lost. There is a whole array of help available to alter the course of the disease, and it is possible to achieve levels of oral and systemic health that were, perhaps, inconceivable and unachievable just a few years ago. This information will be covered in Chapters 7 and 8, but below are some warning signs that might indicate the presence of gum disease.

Signs and Symptoms of Periodontal Disease

- Puffy, red, or swollen gums (swollen gums can be nearly purple, even bluish);

- Bleeding gums (healthy gums *do not* bleed);
- Loose teeth (bone loss and inflammation can loosen teeth);
- Shiny gums (normal gums aren't shiny);
- Changes in the way dental appliances fit (something has moved, not usually the appliance);
- Mouth sores (they need to be checked because, just as a blister or sore isn't normal on the arm, neither is it in the mouth);
- Bad breath (halitosis can be a prominent sign of gum disease);
- A high-sensitivity CRP test reading showing CRP to be elevated (such a reading is regarded as pathological[3]).

CRP TESTS

CRP is a blood test that measures CRP in milligrams (mg) per liter (L), or CRP mg/L (CRP may be reported in different units by your lab). CRP levels of less than 1 mg/L represent a low risk for heart disease, and readings between 1–3 mg/L indicate an average risk for cardiovascular disease. CRP levels of 3 mg/L or higher put people in the high-risk group.[4]

While any elevation of CRP can have serious health consequences, a recent dental study reports that CRP becomes a risk factor for cardiovascular disease, peripheral vascular disease, and stroke at levels of 1.34 mg/L and above.[5]

Please note that although a high-sensitivity CRP test isn't routinely ordered by dentists, either as a diagnostic tool or as a means of monitoring treatment, it should be, because it is a marker that can be tracked. Perhaps more dentists will request this blood test for their patients in the future, but for now, you can request it yourself. If your dentist isn't willing to order this lab test for you, request it from your physician, and have it done annually, at least. It is a very important test, and you need to know your score. High CRP levels can correctly predict a future clotting event, sometimes as much as eight years in advance.

It is never a good idea to diagnose your own disease, but if you do have any of the above signs and symptoms, you should make an appointment with your dentist or periodontist to get a definitive diagnosis. When I suspect periodontal disease, one in-office test I perform is to take my finger and push the gum tissue right where the gum meets the tooth to see if any blood or pus appears. I often get quite a bit of both, along with their odors. While I'm not suggesting you diagnose yourself by pushing on your own gum margins, pus and blood expressed in this manner is a sure sign of a serious health problem for which prompt professional attention is advised.

Finally, and this is based on the current literature as well as my own observations over the last thirty years, the odds are nearly 95 percent that gum disease will show up if there is a careful, complete examination of the mouth and teeth. A competent, concerned dentist can diagnose this for you, so I encourage you to glean all you can from this book, and find someone you trust to help minimize, or even eliminate, periodontal disease as a factor in your life. It's a serious disease, and by applying the appropriate health-enhancing information in this book, in combination with competent and timely periodontal therapy, you will have little reason to worry about gum disease as a continuing health risk in your life.

3

Exploring Inner Space—The Sulcus

A sulcus is defined as a deep, narrow furrow in tissue or an organ, which in dentistry translates to the space between the tooth and the gum tissue, measuring from the edge of the gum (the gingiva, or gingival crest) to where it attaches to the tooth root (the periodontal ligament). See Figure 3.1.

That space between the teeth and the gum tissue—the sulcus—is one that few people outside of dentistry give much thought to, but inside the profession, it is very important. As a practicing dentist, I frequently work in the sulci (plural of "sulcus") and occasionally find myself agonizing over one sulcus. There is even a specialty in dentistry (periodontics) that is primarily concerned with the sulcus, and it is important to monitor what goes on in it because your appearance, your breath, your teeth, your health, even your life itself, can depend on what's going on in all the sulci in your mouth.

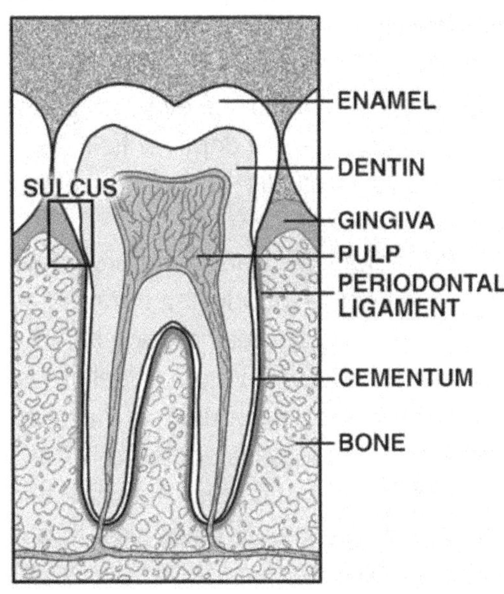

Figure 3.1. The Sulcus with Healthy Tooth and Oral Tissue

For robust gum health and fresh breath, as well as the control of oral factors affecting systemic health, the battle is under the gums, in the sulci of each and every one of us fortunate enough to have teeth (the dentate). The edentulous (toothless) do not have gum disease, since their teeth and associated sulci are gone. However, the edentulous frequently have residual systemic effects from the gum disease that was acquired when they did have teeth. To make this clear to you, let me take you on a tour, a dentist's view of all kinds of sulci, so you will have a much better understanding of what goes on there and why the care of your sulci by you and your dental healthcare professionals is critical to your health. (In preparation for the tour, you may refer to Figure 3.1 for a blueprint of what a sulcus looks like.)

First, we will suit up with a mask and gloves, then reach for a probe (a sulcus-measuring device), and use a little mirror, mostly to keep things out of the way, such as the tongue and cheeks that hang over the sulci we are going to inspect. In order to get a really good view, I'll lend you a pair of operating telescopes just like mine. You wear them like glasses, and everything you see will be magnified approximately four times. When we get into the examination room, we'll plug your fiberoptic cable into your light source and bring it up to its highest intensity. That way, you'll be able to see everything exceedingly well, without shadows, and with an excellent depth of field. You may also be interested to learn that we will actually be peering down into some sulci and looking around.

But before we start, there are a few dos and don'ts to observe on the tour. Prior to introducing our male patient, I must let you know that you are going to be seeing some things for the very first time while dealing with a live patient who has feelings and sensibilities we must respect, and who may be nervous. You may also notice that our probe releases some very unpleasant odors from the sulci. Our patient will never be uncomfortable, but he may not know this. So, while on tour, please don't ask any questions. I'll guide you through what we are seeing as our patient listens because it's critically important to gently educate him about his condition while I am determining what can be done to improve his health. I may ask you to use your mirror to hold his tongue or cheeks back because, as we are inspecting the depths of his sulci, I will also be using an intraoral TV camera to help our patient see, about twenty times larger than life, what we are all seeing on the TV monitor that will be right in front of him. By the way, if any of this bothers you and you feel the need to leave the room, that's perfectly understandable. Just be very careful when you get up; Michelle will unplug your fiberoptic cable and remove your telescopes. You don't even want to know how much these cost, so we don't want to break anything. Whether you stay or not, we'll cover any questions you might have later, once the patient has gone. For now, let me give you a little background on the patient while Michelle seats him in Room 4.

Michelle has taken a full series of digital x-rays on our patient, and I have already reviewed them in my office, but we'll pull them up on the monitor and go over them with the patient after we've completed the periodontal examination; you can see them then. It's easy to demonstrate things on x-rays that are fifteen inches tall, as they will be on the monitor, so you will not have to squint to see the details as you might with little radiographic films. Additionally, thirty minutes ago, my other assistant Tracy gave our patient a measure of protection from the inflammation we will be inducing when we conduct our examination; she gave him three 500 mg chewable vitamin C tablets. This is actually a first-aid recommendation for symptoms of a heart attack[1]; vitamin C is anti-inflammatory and has been shown to dilate blood vessels, so it seems prudent to use it as a preventive measure to help keep inflammation down during our periodontal examination. Michelle has also placed some very effective, eye-protective dark glasses on our patient to shield his eyes from our lights and keep out anything that might otherwise get into his eyes. It's a comfortable and considerate precaution we always take.

Our virtual patient is a thirty-eight-year-old man named Bif (although a fictitious character, he is representative of what is seen in dental offices frequently enough to be a realistic example for our tour). Bif works six days a week as sales manager for the busiest car dealership in town, a job that stresses him to the max, he says. His wife made the appointment for him because his front teeth are dirty and he has a continuous problem with bad breath. Except for being fifty pounds overweight and having joint pains in his hips and knees, Bif claims to have no significant health problems. He does not have a primary care physician and has not had a medical checkup or physical since joining the Air Force as a teenager. Among other things, this leaves both Bif and me in the dark about several critical indicators of his health or any potentially lethal underlying conditions that would show up in blood and urine tests. Bif says he does not take any prescription drugs, but does smoke two packs of cigarettes a day, and admits to drinking "more alcohol than I should." His temperature is slightly elevated at 99.0°F, compared to the norm of 98.6°F.

His last dental visit was ten years ago to have a wisdom tooth removed on the upper left, which "didn't heal right," he said. His oral healthcare efforts include using a hard toothbrush to brush twice a day sometimes, but usually just once, using a popular tartar-control toothpaste. He also carries an alcohol-based mouthwash with him and uses it about every thirty minutes to mask his bad breath. Bif's dental complaints consist of having sore teeth once in a while, and his main concern is to have his teeth cleaned and get something done about his breath. His wife has declined his request to join him in the room, and we are about to begin our tour. Ready?

With all of us in the room, including Bif, we introduce ourselves and briefly review Bif's concerns about his teeth. We also briefly review his health history, not just to confirm what we already know, but perhaps to uncover other factors that could aid our efforts to improve his health. I also take a few moments to reconfirm that we are going to be gathering some information about his condition today, that it will be painless and that, with his permission, I'd like to describe my findings verbally as I go along (asking permission is critical, and since you're in the room with us, you'd just be observing if I couldn't describe things as we go). Bif understands that we will be exploring his sulci with a little measuring instrument marked in millimeters, and recording the numbers on a periodontal chart that can be seen on the monitor. He understands that any readings over 3, or any signs of bleeding, pus, or swelling are not good. He is also aware that healthy teeth should not be loose or covered in tartar, nor should the sulci be covered in plaque. Because of Bif's health and habit history, we're going to be particularly attentive in checking for all this, and more.

Bif has relaxed just a little bit, so we are going to begin our sulci (periodontal) assessment by probing first on the upper right, very gently, next to a molar that shows quite a bit of toothbrush abrasion and recession. On the monitor, Bif can see that his tissue color is fairly good (not red and swollen) on the cheek side of his upper right first molar, number three. When we measure it, he can also see that he has 4 mm of root exposed. Then when I gently slide the probe into the sulcus about mid-tooth, I can feel that the root is smooth, with no tartar deposits; my probing depth is only 1 mm (5 mm is recorded since 4 mm recession plus a 1 mm sulcus depth equals 5 mm). Unfortunately, I can also feel into the furcation, the space between the roots of multi-rooted teeth, which is not a good sign. The good news is, there's no bleeding and no odor, but the tooth has become moderately mobile due to grinding (bruxism) and loss of supporting bone. Bif doesn't know it, but his toothbrush is causing gum recession and root damage as he literally grinds the gum down with a toothbrush that is too hard, and his tooth-grinding isn't helping matters since it overstresses an already weakened tooth.

The second sulcus we are going to explore, right behind the upper right front tooth in tooth number eight, looks very angry. We are going to probe all around the tongue side (the lingual or palatal surface), into the sulcus of this number eight tooth. On the monitor, Bif can see how red and swollen this tissue is. I gently insert the probe straight up under the gum tissue, and keep it right next to the tooth, right into its wide-open sulcus, and find almost no resistance from the very soft tissue. The probe goes past 5 mm under the gum margin, and the root feels very rough and irregular because the tip of the probe is contacting large chunks of subgingival calculus (tartar under the gums). I'm not even at the bottom of the sulcus, yet there's little or no resistance to the probe and we already have considerable bleeding, with just a little pus. While it is painless, there is profuse bleeding. Michelle applies pressure to the area with gauze to control the bleeding, and we wait. Bif is watching this on the monitor as well. Finally, I measure this sulcus to be 8 mm deep, and we record this, as well as the pus and bleeding. It is evident that Bif packs food into this space, just as he does on all his upper front teeth. His upper front teeth have long since moved forward, so his lower front teeth actually bite on the gum margins right over the sulci, allowing the damaging process to accelerate. With a little finger pressure on this tooth, it moves in and out rather easily, perhaps as much as 1 mm each way.

We've checked just two sulci so far (I should explain that sulcus depths can vary from shallow to deep on the same tooth), but it becomes obvious that other measurements around Bif's front teeth would most likely reveal probing depths of perhaps 3–4 mm on the facial (lip) side, with deeper readings between the teeth and on the tongue side. Bif's front teeth are very stained from cigarette smoke, and the gum tissue in front of these teeth has a dull, lifeless appearance, most probably due to the toxic affects of his smoking and his constant use of alcoholic mouthwash. (His gum tissue is subjected to a smoke stream about forty times a day—two packs—and it never has a chance to completely rid itself of the residual surface toxins adhering to it.) Alcohol, especially the 40- to 60-proof mouthwashes commonly available, exert damage to soft tissue in direct proportion to the strength of the mouthwash and the time it is in contact with oral tissues. So the twenty-plus times per day that Bif swishes with his mouthwash could be a total of ten or fifteen minutes of contact daily. This is obviously not conducive to improving his gum tissue health, although it does mask his mouth odor with an even stronger odor.

Bif's examination has barely begun, and it is already apparent that his mouth and his overall health are in serious trouble. Let's check tooth number fifteen, Bif's upper left second molar. As we observe the gum tissue covering the bone on the cheek side of this tooth, which extends toward the front of his mouth about halfway over the root of the tooth in front of number fifteen, we can see a glistening bump about half the size of a small grape (this area would usually be hard and smooth, and any pressure here would be comfortable for the patient). The shiny distended tissue feels just like a small water balloon, and too much pressure would be painful, so we're gentle in our examination of this pus-filled mass.

We are most likely observing either an abscess created by Bif's gum disease and bone loss, or an infection resulting from a dead nerve in one or both of the upper left molars. Either way, I am not going to probe in an area of acute infection, as it is too dangerous for the patient. Remember that acute infection can elevate normal clot-inducing C-reactive-protein levels a thousandfold, and probing could further increase CRP levels, as well as spread infection; so when I see a situation similar to the one affecting Bif on the upper left, it generally means look but don't touch. The x-ray of this periapical area (around the root tips), shows virtually no bone around the root of tooth number fifteen, and this bone loss extends back to one of the roots of the three-rooted molar, number fourteen, which also has no bone around it. Gentle finger pressure on number fifteen shows it to be very mobile, confirming the lack of bone support, which the x-ray revealed. Number fifteen is depressible as well, going down when pushed, and back up when the pressure is released. Bif is in serious trouble, and we've only screened a few of the upper sulci for signs of disease. While it should be obvious that tooth number fifteen can't be saved, my sense is that he has more serious health considerations to pay attention to.

We put Bif in a more upright position to facilitate our examination of his teeth and gums on the lower arch, and proceed to slide our probe through the thick layer of plaque obscuring the sulcus on the cheek side (buccal surface) of number nineteen, a lower left first (six year) molar. This molar is two-rooted, one in front and one in back that are of approximately equal length. When a tooth has two or more roots, the space between the roots where they join the tooth is called "furcation." In a periodontally healthy state, bone will normally cover all of the roots as well as completely fill the space between them. But in Bif's case, the probe goes clear into, and under, the furcation and clear through to the tongue side of the tooth. The probe also created an escape route for approximately ½ cc of very odorous pus. Since it's draining anyway, I put a little finger pressure over the area in an attempt to get out gently as much pus as possible while I'm examining this area, which should make it feel better for Bif.

While Bif has a through-and-through "furcation involvement," the periapical x-ray of the area shows that at least three-quarters of each root is covered in bone. Bif needs some good news; while not great, the prognosis for the lower left teeth, and the possibility of achieving healthy sulci, is certainly better than for the upper left, where extraction of number fifteen is the only option. Probing a diseased sulcus such as this one reveals a wide space that's spongy, or "boggy" as it is sometimes described. (As a reminder, healthy sulci are firm, shallow, and tight, and there's no bleeding when probed.)

The lower front teeth will be examined next and, since gum disease and recession has exposed at least 4–5 mm of the roots of his four lower front teeth, considerable supporting bone has been lost. The two middle teeth are very mobile, but those adjacent to them are slightly firmer. A gentle probing of the sulcus in the front and middle of number twenty-five, the lower right central incisor, reveals a reading of 4 mm, and I am not forcing the probe to go deeper. The left central, number twenty-four, probes similarly. Both teeth reveal slow but definite bleeding. The gum tissue in front of these teeth is dull in appearance. While the gum tissue at the sulcus is not dull, it is slightly pulled away from the teeth, and there appears to be a bluish-greenish color down in the sulcus, next to the tooth.

Any attempt to probe either sulcus on the tongue side of these lower front teeth would be impossible. Bif has such extensive brownish black tartar (calculus) deposits on the tongue side of all six of his lower front teeth that the gums are literally covered up, with no sulci visible (dentists call this a calculus bridge). A review of the periapical x-ray of the lower anterior region shows a very large semicircle of bone loss involving the lower six front teeth, with the root tips (apices) of the two middle ones appearing to sit on top of the bone. There is *no* bone holding these two teeth in, only gum tissue, and the hard deposits encasing them on the tongue side are probably all that has kept these teeth from falling out. The bone loss and hard-deposit pattern seen here is consistent with what is frequently observed in smokers. Tobacco smoke is very toxic to gum tissue, and Bif will be strongly counseled concerning this habit when we discuss his treatment and home-care programs. Whether my patients want to stop tobacco habits or not, I'm with them all the way, but it is a great feeling to be able to help someone successfully kick the tobacco habit.

The last sulci we're going to evaluate by probing are on the lower right. Normally, I would check the two bicuspids (numbers twenty-eight and twenty-nine), but they are missing, and apparently have been for quite some time. The gum tissue over the ridge, all that remains in this toothless area, is atrophied and thin, except directly in the front of the next tooth back, the lower right first molar (number thirty). With both bicuspids gone, all three molars in this quadrant have been allowed to tip toward the front of the mouth, resembling the slanted brick patterns I've seen outlining flowerbeds and sidewalks; they are at about a thirty-degree angle off vertical. This mesial tipping has pushed Bif's gum tissue up the front of the first molar, creating a rounded gum margin at the sulcus, which is under the overhanging tooth and covered in plaque and debris. Feeling our way into the sulcus with the probe reveals a 9 mm probing depth with considerable bleeding and a little pus, as well as rough, hard deposits on the root.

Lower molars almost always have two root canals in the front root, one on the tongue side, and the other on the cheek side. With this tooth, number thirty, it's easy to detect that the groove on the front of the root is quite deep. (Cut in half horizontally, the root would have the same shape as the number eight.) Probing at the furcation on the cheek side of number thirty reveals a distinct furcation involvement since the probe goes all the way to where the roots divide, but it is not a through-and-through situation as it was on the other side. There is, not surprisingly, bleeding at this site as well. This is recorded, and the probing depth of 6 mm is noted as well.

While Bif's gum-health exam isn't over quite yet—we still need to let him know he was a really great patient and arrange to see him soon to discuss our findings and recommendations—I want to make sure you're doing all right at this point. I don't want to assume that you understand just how seriously ill this gentleman is, nor do I want you to get the impression that all we need to be concerned about is getting his mouth cleaned up and his oral home care tuned up, like getting him to brush better and floss effectively. While Bif is purely a fictitious character made up for demonstration purposes, his health history and his serious periodontal disease depict a distressingly common situation that presents quite a number of problems.

It is apparent that Bif is very much at risk for cardiovascular disease, at a minimum. He obviously has severe periodontal disease, in addition to other factors that predispose him to cardiovascular disease—including his two-pack-a-day smoking habit, his being fifty pounds overweight, his high-stress, six-day-a-week job, and his age.

After learning what you have about the correlation between mouth disease and systemic disease, then taking this tour, does periodontal disease look like it's a problem that affects only the mouth? Or is it now apparent that with perhaps twenty-five teeth exposed to as many as 400 different types of oral microorganisms, there's every chance Bif has a serious systemic infection that can possibly threaten several organ systems in his body, and even cause death? If you can see that a seriously diseased mouth is potentially affecting the whole body—the brain, heart, joints, lungs, and more—then you're beginning to see why I am so concerned about this serious health issue.

One recently published study in the *Journal of Periodontology* (September 2001) clearly established that periodontal infections contribute to elevated systemic CRP levels. In this study, elevated levels of CRP were evident in patients with infection from subgingival periodontal pathogens (microorganisms that can cause disease), while elevated CRP was not a significant factor in the healthy controls. The study noted not only the positive correlation between periodontal disease and elevated CRP levels, but also considered that periodontal disease was a possible underlying pathway between periodontal disease and the observed higher risk for cardiovascular disease in these patients.

In another, even more recent study, the participants had blood tests done before and after chewing gum lightly, fifty times on each side, to determine if just chewing gum could elevate circulating levels of proinflammatory components such as endotoxins (toxins of internal origin—harmful bacteria, for example—found in microorganisms). Blood tests were done on the test subjects before and after chewing gum. In those with periodontal disease, such as Bif had, it was found that the blood levels of endotoxins were significantly higher in those after chewing gum than they were before. Before chewing, these levels showed an incidence of positive endotoxemia to be 6 percent, while after chewing gum it rose to 24 percent. The conclusion was that "gentle mastication is able to induce the release of bacterial endotoxins from oral origin into the bloodstream, especially when patients have severe periodontal disease. This finding suggests that a diseased periodontium can be a major and underestimated source of chronic, or even permanent release of bacterial pro-inflammatory components into the bloodstream."[2]

The real challenge here is that patients like Bif do have an extremely serious, even life-threatening, illness, but they have the perception that it's just bleeding gums or something on a par with having a cold. From our tour, it is obvious that Bif has severe periodontal disease; it is exceedingly likely that he has highly elevated CRP levels, positive endotoxemia; and as suggested by the two studies mentioned above, he is in a category that puts him at a greater risk for cardiovascular disease. Bif is in trouble, and his situation is, unfortunately, seen in a distressingly high percentage of adult patients.

Everything considered, even if the Bifs out there go ahead and have treatment, such as scaling and root planing, or required surgical procedures, once their treatment is completed, they assume they are cured.

Since we've already talked about gum disease being a systemic infection, and not just a problem that is somehow compartmentalized in the mouth, it is imperative for dentists and patients alike to begin viewing this disease as the serious infection it is. We must also begin taking a serious look at different methods, materials, and techniques that are used effectively to combat what is essentially an inflammatory, infectious process. The relatively recent proliferation of studies and articles about the periodontal-systemic disease connection appearing in our professional journals gives me hope that this serious health issue is finally going to become recognized for what it is. And from that, I'm hopeful that much more will be forthcoming about what patients need to do to become far healthier.

In the meantime, there are still a considerable number of problems that must be examined, and changed, before any meaningful improvement in the periodontal-systemic disease situation can be addressed by the public and the dental profession. Ironically, it was physicians, not dentists, who originally initiated my research into CRP, and it is physicians and other non-dental health professionals who have authored a number of books with chapters on periodontal disease, outlining safe, effective methods to combat this serious situation. Why then are so many dentists and physicians dragging their feet about this critical health issue? Maybe they will begin to jump on the bandwagon now that CRP is in the news as a major cause of heart attacks and strokes, as well as other serious health issues; now that there are articles about how its reduction and control figure so prominently in maintaining a strong, healthy mouth and better overall health. That dentistry has begun to scrutinize this situation more intensely bodes well, but so far, dentistry and oral care hasn't resulted in robust oral health *or* robust systemic health. If you just look at the incidence of periodontal disease, heart attacks, and strokes, you get a sense of the magnitude of this public-health failure. We are losing the war and we need to look elsewhere. Fortunately, much of what we need for better results is already known and available, and is presented here for your consideration and potential benefit, should you decide you need or want to make changes in your own health program.

What about the dental procedures Bif needs to have done in the office? We're going to leave that alone because the focus of this book is on what he (or you) needs to do for himself, not what a dentist needs to do for him once there is a problem. But my experience tells me that, without taking advantage of any of the information in this book, Bif has an extraordinarily grim prognosis. Do you think he'll make the changes necessary to live a lot longer? Let's recommend that he see a knowledgeable physician for a complete history and physical, all necessary lab tests, including a high-sensitivity CRP analysis. Then we'll be better able to help Bif address his serious health issues. He's at a fork in the road. Dead ahead lies continued illness, or he can make a turn toward a much healthier life. Hopefully, we have given him the information he needs to make a good decision. You were there with us, and I certainly hope you enjoyed the tour.

4

From Health to Disease—How to Gum-up the Works

This chapter discusses the progression of a normal molar and its associated structures, including its sulcus, from a state of health to one of serious periodontal—and therefore systemic—disease. Figures 4.1 through 4.5 illustrate this movement by showing a typical lower right first molar that eventually loses its supporting structure of bone and is, therefore, lost to disease. Just this one molar alone could exact a severe toll on the health of the person in whose mouth it resides, and since periodontal disease is seldom confined to just one tooth, the cumulative effect of several infected teeth can be, and often is, severe.

Let's begin our trip with a healthy tooth and oral tissue, as illustrated by Figure 3.1 (see page 23). This figure shows the protective layer of gum tissue surrounding the first molar. This tissue is doing its job of protecting the body from infection, toxins, and other potential injury by keeping out the approximately 400 types of microorganisms that live, multiply, and die mainly in the sulcus. In addition, the gum tissue lining the sulcus protects it from the dead skin cells (desquamated epithelial cells) that slough off into it from the gum-tissue wall. Food debris forced under the gum tissue can also present a problem, as can the act of consuming a typical diet with the chewing required to process food for proper digestion, which puts stress and abrasions on the healthy gum tissue.

In reference to frank (obvious) periodontal disease only, the molar and its underlying bone will remain healthy as long as the gum-tissue barrier remains intact, which is not an easy thing to do since the sulcus is a potential cesspool of microorganisms and debris under the gums. However, as long as the sulcular tissue lining the sulcus wall remains healthy and intact, the microorganisms, toxins, and other unhealthy elements will stay out of the body. But how do you know when your gums are healthy? You know because healthy gums do not bleed when brushed, flossed, or stimulated by toothpicks or other devices designed to facilitate cleaning the sulcus under the gums.

Keep in mind that gum disease affects from 75 to 95 percent of the adult population. Figure 4.1 depicts gingivitis and its associated inflammation, indicating the beginning of gum disease and its potentially serious systemic effects.

Gingivitis is a condition in which the gums are inflamed, swollen, tender, and discolored (usually red, and sometimes very red). The causes of gingivitis vary from poor oral hygiene or smoking to harsh oral health efforts, such as the use of hard toothbrushes or overzealous flossing. Additionally, hormonal or metabolic disturbances, such as pregnancy or diabetes, can lead to an increased risk of gingivitis. Ongoing studies of periodontal disease show that the causes of the disease can vary, but several facts emerge when there is a diagnosis of gingivitis. First, gingivitis is

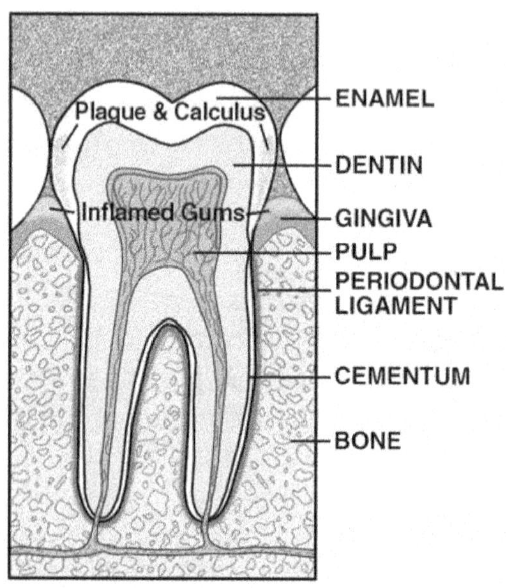

Figure 4.1. Gingivitis (inflammation of the gums)

the initial stage of a potentially destructive process that leads to periodontal disease, and perhaps even more ominously, gingivitis is where inflammation makes its appearance as a potentially harmful systemic condition with potentially deleterious health effects down the road.

In spite of the actual health challenges presented by gingivitis, the common perception is that this condition is just bleeding gums and, therefore, of little consequence. Dr. Larry Emmott probably said it best when, in referring to a study of more than 50,000 people in four countries that verified the connection between periodontal disease and heart disease, he stated that he was very impressed by research that "could serve to wake up a society that is at risk of becoming dangerously blasé about periodontal disease."[1]

Dr. Emmott was being gentle in his assessment of the collective attitude concerning periodontal disease. Mine would be that people have always been dangerously blasé about this potentially fatal disease and, for the most part, continue to be unconcerned to this day. (You constitute an exception since you wouldn't be reading this if gum disease were of no interest or concern to you.) So, when the gum infection called gingivitis is present, we are dealing with a potentially serious condition that could be the gateway to a *more* serious condition if it isn't reversed at this stage.

The good news is that gingivitis is almost always reversible, but it doesn't go away on its own. Unfortunately, people frequently resort to toxic toothpastes and mouthwashes in an attempt to bring their gingivitis infection under control; in Chapter 5, you will learn that using products that specifically warn the user to call the poison control center immediately if their child, or others, ingests some of the toothpaste or mouthwash is not conducive to regaining health.

At fifteen, soon after my kindly dentist informed me of my gingivitis, I had my first and only experience with a mouthwash that must have been the prototype for firewater. I used it just once. I also used a natural bristle brush that was exceedingly hard—but I didn't use it for long. Something in the back of my pre-dental mind told me something wasn't quite right with my tools and techniques. Now, four decades later, we still have firewater and hard brushes and I'm still investigating products. I'll have more to say about this later, but delicate oral tissues need some help in order to heal a gingivitis inflammation and its potential consequences; harsh toxic products do not provide that help. If gingivitis is present, it must be dealt with aggressively by having health professionals and their patients pay attention to this problem and do something safe and effective about it.

You will learn how to stop gingivitis effectively in later chapters, but for now we're going to allow the infectious gingivitis in Figure 4.1 to progress to early periodontitis (see Figure 4.2).

Early periodontitis represents the progression of gingivitis to a more deep-seated infection characterized by bone loss and considerably increased levels of inflammation. Sulcus probing will go to a depth of 4–5 mm due to bone loss and swelling, and bleeding and pus will frequently show up with the probing. Gentleness is required when probing because these infected tissues will be very tender. This stage of periodontal disease begins to trigger my concern about the potentially serious side effects of CRP and, depending upon the age and sex of my patient, my advice will vary.

When men at this stage of the disease are at least in their late twenties, I begin to become concerned because this is when men who were thought to be perfectly healthy start to die of unexplained heart attacks.

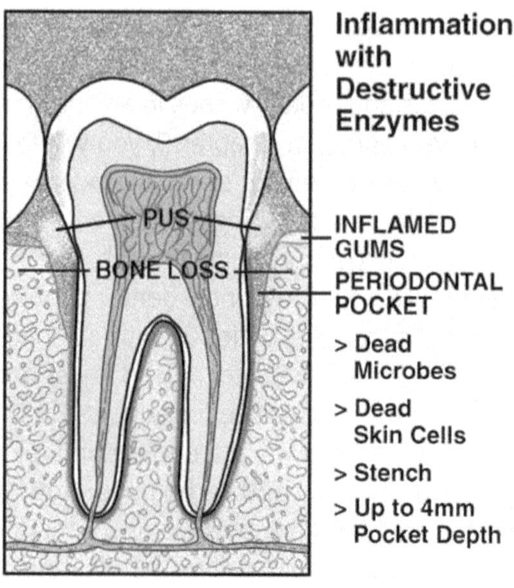

Figure 4.2. Early Periodontitis

I am just as concerned about women, but they seem to have a cardioprotective mechanism at play until they are perimenopausal, which usually begins in their mid-forties. Occasionally, however, women also die unexpectedly of heart attacks well before menopause, so I recommend aggressive treatment of this disease, regardless of age or sex.

Figure 4.2 illustrates a sulcus that is deep *and* wide. To explain how the systemic effects of gum disease are dose related, I will ask you to imagine that the gum tissue wrapped around the molar in Figure 4.2 is unwrapped. How much surface area of infected, inflamed tissue would that be? If we measured 5 mm deep and estimated about 40 mm around, and then laid this out and looked at it, there might be from one-third to a square inch of infected, inflamed tissue. Since this raw infected tissue is no longer a barrier, microorganisms and inflammatory components (creating CRP) have nothing to stop them from entering the circulatory system to potentially wreak havoc upon the health of this person.

Multiply this infected area by six, or even twelve, teeth with probing depths of 5 mm all the way around each tooth. If that infected tissue were laid out, it could measure from two to four square inches. While this might be hard to visualize, the mere fact that we can't see this ulcerated, infected tissue doesn't mean the person isn't affected by it. He or she is very much affected (infected), and the more surface area involved, the bigger the problem. That is what is meant by dose related. In full-blown gum disease, if all the affected gum tissue around a full complement of teeth were laid out, it would be equivalent to the entire back of your hand. Further, imagine there are twenty-four to twenty-eight teeth imbedded in the back of your hand, all with the same inflammation and infection we saw when we toured Bif's mouth. Visualize this painless process out in the open and it wouldn't be hard for the person to understand that serious illness was involved, would it? This unpleasant mental picture graphically illustrates what the body has to deal with in terms of a systemic infection with loads of inflammation and elevated CRP. Since processes that may be out of sight can still wreak havoc on your health, I hope this illustration has helped you visualize the sheer extent of the problem that is, for the most part, incapable of showing itself.

Before any periodontal therapy is begun, I recommend getting a high-sensitivity CRP test, because CRP is a marker of the degree of inflammation and the ensuing potential health risk. As you recall, CRP is responsible for quite a number of serious health conditions, including heart attacks and strokes, and the higher the CRP number, the higher the likelihood of a serious problem, so a baseline CRP reading is well-advised before treatment is begun. This is what I do in my practice. Although a pretreatment CRP test isn't even close to mainstream dental practice now, I see it as a logical part of a dental health assessment in the future.

The person with the early periodontitis in Figure 4.2 is potentially in even greater peril if the illness is also systemic, and it gets worse.

The next stage of disease, the moderate periodontitis depicted in Figure 4.3, is a very deep-seated infection, and anyone who comes to me with this condition tends to have a characteristic look and demeanor, but doesn't generally associate any of this with gum disease, or even realize the condition is there. While this stage of periodontal disease is termed "moderate" in dental terms, it is far more serious than that when viewed as a systemic infection.

Anyone with moderate periodontitis is generally going to have considerable redness and swelling in the mouth, usually with a buildup of

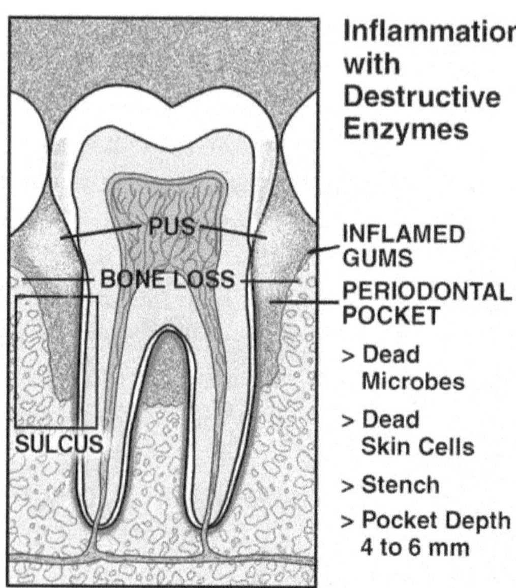

Figure 4.3. Moderate Periodontitis

hard deposits above and below the gum margin, perhaps an unpleasant odor, and possibly several loose teeth. This person will often be dull-eyed, listless and tired, pale to almost jaundiced in appearance, and will admit to being a little blue or depressed, if questioned.

It should come as no surprise that people with moderate periodontitis have been affected by their disease for a considerable length of time, perhaps many years, and are already undergoing treatment by their physicians for some of their conditions. These could include arthritis and rheumatoid arthritis, diabetes, fibromyalgia, high blood pressure, high cholesterol, pulmonary edema, and shortness of breath. Inasmuch as their immune systems can be severely challenged by circulating microorganisms and inflammatory components, such as leukotrienes, proinflammatory cytokines, and prostaglandins, as well as the resultant CRP, it would not be an exaggeration to view such people as very ill, would it? Are you starting to see just how ill people like this really are?

Additionally, people in this category are almost invariably on several prescription medications, many of which carry life-threatening side effects of their own. The statin drugs, for instance, do a marvelous job at reducing cholesterol, but they also dramatically reduce coenzyme Q_{10}, an immune-system stimulant and an antioxidant, which is required for life itself. CoQ_{10} has a number of health-enhancing properties, some dramatic, and studies indicate that its levels are notably reduced in diseased heart and periodontal tissues. (Prescription drugs can be beneficial, even necessary, but, as I mentioned earlier, they were also the number-four cause of death in 2001, with an estimated 265,000 deaths. There are other, safer, effective methods than statins for addressing elevated cholesterol levels, unhealthy HDL/LDL ratios, and low CoQ_{10} levels, which let you take a pass on the adverse side effects.)

It is important to point out again that people are affected by *all* the cumulative inflammation present in their bodies. All inflammation raises CRP levels, so an adult male with arthritis, prostate inflammation, and moderate periodontal disease—not an uncommon combination of ailments—would need some serious help in regaining his health (and there is much that can be done). Anyone with these conditions should not regard them as the result of just getting older, as if these problems were inevitable. They are not, and the individual should know that these conditions exist primarily because he or she did not have the benefit of nutritional regimens and lifestyle choices that may have prevented them in the first place. It is not the scope of this book to go in depth into areas outside of dental health issues, but you should be aware that regimens for periodontal health can, and frequently do, positively affect other health conditions.

It is always a good idea to consult with your personal physician if you have any questions about a periodontal health and wellness program because a review of the recommendations obtained from a number of highly credible medical sources shows that most of the risk lies in doing nothing.[2]

Figure 4.4 illustrates end-stage periodontal disease. As discussed, someone with this level of disease almost invariably has a number of related diseases. It's practically inevitable because *the mouth mirrors the health of the body.*

In this condition, the surface area of the inflamed periodontal tissue in the infected sulci can exceed several square inches. The tissue is neither an effective barrier nor a contributor to health, since its inflammatory components elevate CRP levels.

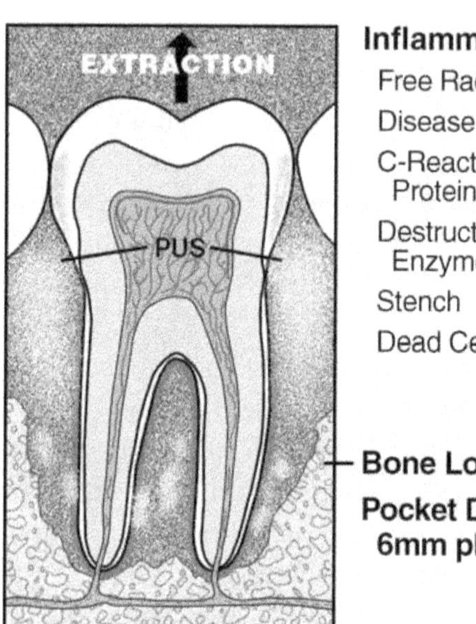

Figure 4.4. Severe Periodontitis

As with the other three stages of periodontal disease depicted in this chapter, professional help is required to treat severe periodontitis effectively. And, although it may not be widely recognized at the present time, the treatment of periodontal disease at this end stage is as risky for the uninformed, unprepared patient as it is for the treating dentist. Any dentist faced with this level of disease should be aware that it can be dangerous to manipulate infected, inflamed tissues in an unprotected patient; by doing so, the dentist may dramatically elevate CRP in periodontal patients who probably already have elevated levels of CRP.[3]

Dentistry Today reports, "As an independent risk factor for cardiovascular disease, high normal levels of CRP are associated with risk of angina, heart attack, and death," and adds that severe infection or inflammation can raise CRP levels to levels 500 times greater than normal.[4] Five hundred times over high normal limits is very risky territory to be in and, as if a 500-fold elevation of CRP weren't enough, consider the additional increase in inflammation when a well-meaning dentist or hygienist starts cleaning the already inflamed, infected sulci using ultrasonic, water-spraying, vibrating tips at the deepest levels of these infected areas. Besides dramatically increasing inflammation, this puts the microorganisms in an almost blenderlike vortex, with a percentage of the debris being forced into the adjacent ulcerated tissue, the sulcular wall labeled "gingiva" in Figure 4.5. When this ultrasonic or hand scaling is done around twelve or fourteen teeth (half a mouth), CRP levels will rise even further, perhaps as much as 300 percent above the pretreatment baseline, according to one double-blind study.

While several theories concerning the connection between periodontal disease and cardiac disease exist, all agree that there *is* some connection. On July 26–27 of 2001, the American Dental Association (ADA) held the first symposium ever to discuss and provide perspectives on the periodontal-systemic disease connection. The first installment in a planned series was titled "Taking Oral Health to Heart: Exploring the Interrelationship Between Oral and Cardiovascular Disease."[5]

Potential mechanisms of association were reported, suggesting that there is evidence from studies to support the idea that periodontal pathogens have systemic effects that cause the progression of coronary artery disease. Studies showed that *Porphyromonas gingivalis* "can cause platelet aggregation, increase lipids, enhance atheroma formation

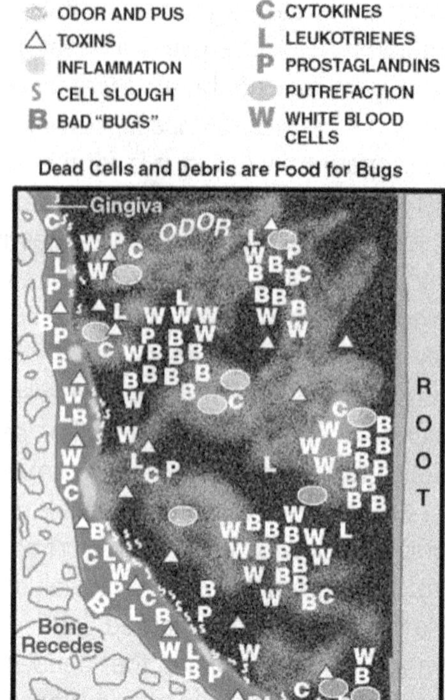

Figure 4.5. Microorganism Battle

and increase calcification." Moreover, at least one study recovered *P. gingivalis* from heart and liver tissue, while others found it in atheromas (clots) and the coronary and carotid endothelium (the innermost lining of arteries). If this theory is correct, it would be very well indeed to keep the sulcular walls intact and acting as a true barrier to keep *P. gingivalis* confined to the mouth, and not circulating throughout the body.

A second possible mechanism is offered by two researchers from The University of North Carolina, epidemiologist Dr. James Beck, Ph.D., and a professor of periodontology, Dr. Steven Offenbacher. They contend that the oral-systemic "association is related to host mechanisms, such as inflammatory response and antibody production." According to Dr. Beck, "The clinical signs of periodontal disease are not a specific indication of systemic effects," stating further that clinical signs of periodontal disease may only *represent* the relationship between periodontal disease and coronary heart disease. "People can have the organisms and the infection that cause periodontal disease, but not have clinical signs of the disease. We believe it's the host's inflammatory response that causes the disease," stated Dr. Beck. Supporting this theory of association, Dr. Offenbacher said, "researchers are finding a correlation between the depth of the periodontal pocket and the levels of some of these inflammatory mediators."[6]

If this association is correct, and it's my firm conviction that it is, helpful solutions are at hand. It is my opinion that there is an anti-inflammatory regimen that could prevent either, or both, diseases and could even reverse existing disease to some degree (this regimen is not drug-based, has an exceptional degree of safety, and has been very effective for many of my patients). Inflammation is finally being implicated as a very real problem, not only in periodontal disease, but in systemic disease as well.

Dr. Robert Genco, chairman of the SUNY–Buffalo Department of Oral Biology, also reported support for the role of inflammatory mediators in perio-cardiac associations. Dr. Genco was the person who observed that CRP levels increase up to 500 times in the presence of severe infection or inflammation. He also reported that periodontal patients had higher than normal levels of CRP and that a periodontal procedure performed in combination with the patient taking a nonsteroidal anti-inflammatory resulted in decreased CRP, while scaling and root planing alone "appear to have the opposite effect" (they elevate CRP).[7]

Go back to Figure 4.5 and imagine that the inflamed, infected tissue depicted was all torn up around twenty-eight teeth as a natural result of a deep-cleaning procedure. It should be obvious that, with all the microorganisms introduced into the circulatory system by deep cleaning, and with the dramatic increase in inflammation caused by the procedure, the whole process represents a serious physiological assault on the person receiving the therapy. It is risky business for the unprotected patient.

There are any number of safe and effective things you can do to improve your oral and systemic health, as well as increase the margin of safety during periodontal procedures. These primarily involve using a very wide range of nutritional elements, such as antioxidants, vitamins, and minerals, many of which are exceedingly effective anti-inflammatories. Additionally, there's a potent Cox-II inhibitor, Zincosamine, that would be worthy of some professional consideration because, in a study, it was shown to specifically neutralize the substances known to elevate CRP levels.[8] At the very least, anyone with arthritis would likely get relief using it, as most in the study did.

From the disease progression depicted in Figures 4.1–4.5, we've seen that, while the molar tooth is the central part of the picture, systemic disease caused by either inflammation or microorganisms entering the body through the diseased sulcular tissues is clearly the *BIG* picture. Chapter 5 will deal with the pitfalls and inadequacies of home care as it is taught and practiced at the present time and, with your knowledge of the sulcus—gained from the tour of our accommodating patient, Bif—I believe you will clearly understand why the methods and materials most people use for home care these days fall short in helping them achieve oral or systemic health. I don't know about you, but I'm ready to take on gum disease and start fighting back.

5

Toxic Toothpaste and Scary Mouthwash

At the end of the last chapter, I said I was ready to take on gum disease and start fighting back. So with that in mind, I reread the labels on commonly used toothpaste and mouthwash bottles, and they reinforced my belief that these would not be my weapons of choice for serious health problems. I've seen the damage these toxic products can do—the burning red mouths, the cheek tissue sloughing off in sheets, the tongues so red and swollen the patients could barely speak, much less swallow—and I don't like it. All that these affected people had done was use the same toothpastes and mouthwashes you are probably using right now, so-called therapeutic products, which end up being pathological for some. In this chapter, I intend to tackle these products and give you some insight into why there's so much disease out there, including cancer and death, from using these off-the-shelf oral health products.

As you study all the warnings and facts concerning the harmful ingredients in the oral health products some people are hurting themselves with every day, please realize that the prevailing idea generally promoted by sales reps is, while a small amount of toxic stuff *is* in the products they proffer, there's not very much, so it's not a big deal. Imagine my telling a mother there's a rattlesnake in the petting zoo, but it's just a little one.

Most people select a specific toothpaste or mouthwash for their own particular reasons, perhaps for its color or taste. Maybe they saw an advertisement for a product and thought they might try it based on something mentioned in the ad. Why do you use the toothpaste and mouthwash that's in your cabinet? Could it be that there are some very compelling ads for toothpastes and mouthwashes that purport to provide the user with all sorts of benefits, from fewer cavities to fresher breath and removing more plaque than brushing by itself can accomplish? Only you know why you use what you use.

From my perspective as a dentist, for someone to have a reasonable chance of creating a healthier mouth with their home-care efforts, it would clearly be to their advantage to use products that have known health-enhancing benefits. Since the odds are great that they already have some condition they'd like to heal and not aggravate further, it would also make sense to *avoid* any toothpaste or mouthwash containing substances known to be clearly harmful.

Using safe products also makes sense because oral soft tissues are literally a sponge just waiting to absorb into the body whatever comes in contact with the lips, cheeks, tongue, and throat. Anyone who has ever eaten a hot pepper has experienced just how fast the burning sensation comes on, and how hard it is to get rid of once it has established itself. These hot foods announce themselves so you are aware of what you are doing, but what about substances that are harmful and get absorbed through the oral tissues so quietly that there's no pain? What can be done about those?

In trying to answer this question, let's first review the warnings on a few different pastes and washes, given below, to get an idea just how toxic this situation is. (This list could be a lot longer since dozens of products contain essentially the same toxic ingredients.)

- *Mouthwash.* Warning: Keep out of the reach of children. Do not use in children under six years of age. In case of accidental misuse, seek professional assistance or contact a poison control center immediately. Do not swallow.

- *Mouthwash.* This package for households without young children.

- *Toothpaste.* Do not swallow. Instruct children under six years in good rinsing habits (to reduce swallowing). Supervise children as necessary until capable of using without supervision. Rinse away toothpaste residue after brushing.

- *Toothpaste.* Warning: Use a pea-sized amount and supervise until good habits are established.
- *Toothpaste.* **Warning: Keep out of reach of children under six years of age** (in bold type on box). If more than used for brushing is accidentally swallowed, get medical help right away or contact a poison control center right away. If irritation occurs and persists, discontinue use.

Now, how do we determine if one of our children has swallowed a bit of this swill? If it's in the throat, it could be on its way to the stomach, so do we need to have the poison control center's number at the ready just in case they end up swallowing some? Can't say we weren't warned, can we? The challenge with toothpastes and mouthwashes is to find one *without* these types of warnings.

THE NINE UNTOUCHABLES

While people are free to use what they want, I believe it's a good idea for everyone to know what's in the products we're using for our oral health. Please read the labels on your toothpaste and mouthwash, and see if any of the following ingredients appear. (Warning: I lose my good nature when I ponder products with the following ingredients in them, since none of them are safe to use.)

Triclosan

Triclosan is EPA-registered as a pesticide. This chlorophenol gets high marks as a risk to both humans and the environment. It is in a class of chemicals suspected of causing cancer in humans, and is similar in structure to dioxin, whose toxic effects are measured in parts per trillion (1 drop in 300 Olympic-size swimming pools). Triclosan is a hormone disrupter as well, and can lead to circulatory collapse, cold sweats, and convulsions. Because it is stored in body fat, it can accumulate to toxic levels, which can lead to a number of problems, including brain hemorrhages, heart conditions, kidney damage, and paralysis. Since the oral soft tissues readily absorb whatever is in contact with them (remember the hot pepper), building up triclosan residues in the body could be easily accomplished. Triclosan in your toothpaste anyone?

Propylene Glycol (PG)

Your Chevrolet recognizes propylene glycol as antifreeze, and you probably know that antifreeze has killed many cats and dogs that have lapped it up. PG is used as a wetting agent in toothpaste, but it is so readily absorbed into the skin that the EPA requires anyone working around it to wear goggles and protective clothing. The Material Safety Data Sheet (MSDS) warns against skin contact because PG has systemic consequences, such as brain, kidney, and liver abnormalities. However, no such warning is required on underarm deodorants, toothpastes, or other products containing PG. Does the use of PG in toothpaste, for use in an area where it's readily absorbed, seem logical to you?

Sodium Hydroxide (NaOH)

In high concentration, sodium hydroxide (NaOH), an extremely alkaline substance, destroys protein instantly. In the mouth, it dissolves oral soft tissues, imparting a slick feeling. Dissolving off the protein with NaOH is not the way I want my patients to get clean teeth; dissolving delicate oral tissues isn't going to help them be a better, more competent barrier, is it?

Sodium Lauryl Sulfate (SLS)

Sodium lauryl sulfate (SLS), a ubiquitous detergent and surfactant, which is also used in car washes, engine degreasers, and garage floor cleaners, poses a serious health risk because, like NaOH, it dissolves proteins. Animals exposed to SLS experience diarrhea, eye damage, labored breathing, skin irritation, and even death. When combined with other chemicals, SLS can be transformed into nitrosamines, a potent class of carcinogens. The body retains SLS for up to five days, during which time it may enter and maintain residual levels in the brain, heart, liver, and lungs.

Sodium Laureth Sulfate (SLES)

A toxic substance and close relative of SLS, sodium laureth sulfate (SLES) is known to have similar harmful effects, and is also common in many products used in this country. Both SLES and SLS are used in toothpaste, to make it foam. Given the health risks associated with each of them, do we really need these chemicals just for foam?

Polyethylene Glycol (PEG)

Polyethylene glycol (PEG) is used in cleansers to dissolve oil and grease, and in personal products as a thickener. PEG is a potential carcinogenic substance that, when used on the skin, alters its natural moisture factor, leaving the skin vulnerable to aging and invasion by harmful bacteria. PEG has no logical therapeutic benefit in toothpastes, but it is in quite a number of them.

Alcohol, Isopropyl (SD-40)

SD-40, an alcohol found in a number of toothpastes, is very dehydrating and acts as a carrier, facilitating the entry of other harmful chemicals into your oral soft tissues. On the skin, it promotes premature aging and brown spots. A fatal ingested dose is one ounce or less, and according to *A Consumers Dictionary of Cosmetic Ingredients,* it may cause dizziness, flushing, headaches, mental depression, narcosis, nausea, vomiting, and even coma. As with all the other harmful substances listed, I don't know why SD-40, with its potentially harmful effects, is a common ingredient in toothpaste.

FD&C Color Pigments

FD&C color pigments (Red No. 40, Green No. 5, Blue No. 1, Yellow No. 10, Red No. 30 lake, Yellow No. 10 lake) are all synthetic colors made from coal tar, and animal studies have shown almost all of them to be carcinogenic. Many of these colors contain heavy metal salts, which can accumulate in the body and cause serious health problems. Do toothpastes and mouthwashes really need to be red, blue, green, and yellow? Those coal-tar-derived colors may look nice, but at what cost to the user's health?

Ethanol (Ethyl Alcohol)

Ethanol is the primary component in the majority of mouthwashes, and it has an extraordinary ability to draw moisture out of living cells, noticeably dehydrating tissues. With alcohol contents of nearly 27 percent (54 proof), alcohol-based mouthwashes are known to be a cause of oral cancer for approximately 36,000 users a year (only smokers are more at risk for this form of cancer), and there were approximately 500 deaths in the year 2000 from this form of alcohol ingestion. Of all the ingredients in oral health products, alcohol may be the most harmful. Besides dehydration and the oral cancer risks associated with it, studies show that alcohol dissolves cosmetic fillings. University studies of twelve mouthwashes showed that nine of them degraded or deteriorated cosmetic bonding or cosmetic filling materials. Two of the three that did not harm composites were an alcohol-free mouthwash and a mild alcohol-containing mouthwash. They did not degrade the four tooth-colored filling materials tested (water was used as a control), and the harm to the filling materials was generally proportional to the alcohol content of the mouthwash. With all the known problems and safety issues associated with alcohol-based mouthwashes, common sense dictates that they be avoided, if for no other reason than because they damage excellent (and expensive) cosmetic dentistry.

THE BEST ALTERNATIVES

Now for solutions to the problems posed by harmful oral health products. My first recommendation is to read toothpaste and mouthwash labels to ensure there are *no* harmful ingredients in them. There *are* safe and effective toothpastes and mouthwashes available that offer substantial benefits. While there may be a few commonly available brands I have not used myself, or evaluated in my patients who may have used them, there are a few products I have used extensively, and I recommend them without hesitation. Products can be manufactured from all-natural ingredients, or from synthetic compounds that offer the desired effects. I use and recommend both types to patients every day because I know they are safe and they most definitely work.

The toothpaste and mouthwash I like for myself, and have evaluated in hundreds of patients, is BGSE Mint Toothpaste and BGSE Mint Mouthwash Treatment. BGSE is an abbreviation for *BioEnhanced Grapefruit Seed Extract,* and while grapefruit seed extract is just one of the ingredients, this bioflavonoid offers astonishing oral health benefits. It is an excellent cleanser and is capable of inhibiting a wide variety of microorganisms with no toxicity to the user. I *want* this product, or similar products containing grapefruit seed extract, to stay in contact with my patients' oral soft tissues. Other natural ingredients in the toothpaste include hesperidin, a bioflavonoid required for collagen (the building block of soft tissue, bone, and cartilage) formation, the antioxidants cranberry and willowherb, and MSM (methylsulfonylmethane), which is anti-inflammatory and antimicrobial. As if that weren't enough, green tea, a very potent antioxidant, is also included. While the product manufacturer can't make specific health claims for either the toothpaste or the mouthwash, these products have worked quickly, safely, and effectively for my patients and my family. As with any product or food, there can always be people who exhibit some sensitivity to an ingredient, although I have never seen any of my patients have a problem with either—only beneficial results when they are used properly, and often enough.

It is important to mention that BGSE Mint Mouthwash Treatment and BGSE Mint Toothpaste are not only made from all-natural ingredients, but are also totally organic. Neither have microbiological or chemical contaminants, just pure ingredients, so their potential benefit to the user, as well as their total lack of toxic ingredients, represents a considerable departure from the products most people use now. There are literally hundreds of toothpastes and mouthwashes to choose from, and a few of them really *are* worth using. I have reviewed the ingredients of quite a number of natural toothpastes and mouthwashes, and I am very happy to report that many of them not only did not contain ingredients to avoid (the untouchables), but they did contain ingredients that tell me these companies mean business when it comes to doing something about promoting oral health with their products. Many of the natural toothpastes and mouthwashes I reviewed contained potentially beneficial ingredients such as tea tree oil, aloe vera, CoQ_{10}, Ester C, green tea, chamomile, myrrh, and echinacea, and no harmful ingredients. Jason and Tom's of Maine are two companies offering some products I could very enthusiastically support, and there are many other formulations by literally hundreds of companies that could very well be quite safe and effective. Ultimately, you need to decide for yourself what's best for you, and I hope the information I've provided will help you find something you like that also happens to be safe and effective.

You are most likely to find the products you want at either the smaller health food or nutrition stores, or order online and have them delivered to your home. Most of the bigger food stores and drugstores don't have much to choose from that isn't loaded with untouchables, but I expect them to begin offering better products when consumer preferences indicate that the availability of safe and effective products is expected.

An additional mouthwash I have used for several years and have recommended to patients is a synthetic formulation that is totally safe, alcohol-free, and very effective for cleansing and deodorizing the mouth. Oxyfresh Fresh Mint Mouthrinse with Zinc is a stabilized chlorine dioxide, zinc acetate formulation that literally destroys the odors responsible for bad breath. Research has shown that these odors, specifically volatile sulfur compounds (VSC), are at least partially responsible for activating enzymes that dissolve soft tissue (proteolytic enzymes), so whether this product is used as a mouthwash or as an addition to the water used in oral irrigators, it isn't unusual to observe amazing improvements in oral health. (You might recognize from other sources two VSCs found in the mouth: the sewer gas odor comes from methyl mercaptan, and the rotten egg smell comes from hydrogen sulfide.)

The Oxyfresh company claims only cleansing and deodorizing benefits for this mouthwash, so any other benefits discussed here are based on my clinical observation. Ultimately, fighting gum disease and its systemic consequences is a battle best left to products that will do the job, and while the product lines I've mentioned don't make health claims, as a dentist, my experience observing the results of their use leads me to recommend them.

There is a small, but growing, consumer movement away from harmful products, and toward robust oral health. I hope this movement accelerates considerably in the near future because it is the only option that makes good sense. When enough consumers blatantly reject harmful toothpastes and mouthwashes in favor of safe, effective ones, we could see a shift in what the manufacturers of these products have to offer. Meanwhile, the products mentioned above are available and work well, so leave the toxic toothpastes and scary mouthwashes, the untouchables, on the shelf and find something that supports health rather than compromises it. You can find information on how to acquire these products, as well as thorough instructions for their use, at my website listed in the "Contact Dr. Bonner" section on page 122.

For additional information on the untouchables in personal-care products, go to the expert Linda Chaé.[1] A gentle person, Linda is a major force in the movement to get rid of the untouchables in personal and household products. She has decades of experience in formulating alternative, safe, personal-care products, and has even testified at congressional hearings concerning the harmful ingredients most commercial products contain.

Since almost anything goes right now when it comes to most commercially available product formulations, and I'm not just referring to toothpastes and mouthwashes, I take great care to use safe products myself. I encourage you to do the same, since daily internal and external use of products containing known harmful ingredients carries some health risk, and our goal, after all, is to improve your health.

6

Brushing and Flossing Aren't Enough

The title of this chapter brings to mind something I hear at least every week from a patient who has just been diagnosed with some degree of gum disease, and that is, "I brush and floss every day. I couldn't possibly have gum disease." I can genuinely empathize with patients who didn't know they had a systemic infectious disease with potentially serious health risks, and can easily understand their frustration upon discovering that their conscientious home-care efforts simply weren't capable of keeping them healthy.

Having discussed what goes on under the gums, in the sulcus, we know how important it is to cleanse this space frequently enough to make sure the gum tissue remains a healthy barrier. This isn't easy, especially if you are depending on brushing and flossing to accomplish this important task; you have to consider the sheer volume of food debris, living and dead microorganisms, odors, sloughed-off skin cells, and toxins that can build up around the normal complement of twenty-eight to thirty-two teeth in that space under the gums. In the majority of cases, this stew in the sulcus is the spark that sets off periodontal disease. While not pleasant to think about, all this is toxic waste that contains the rotted remains of literally trillions of dead microorganisms, all producing inflammation and odor that is, for the most part, trapped in the sulcus. This stew can also contain various amounts of dead white blood cells (the cells that fight infection when they are living), with sulcular pus and periodontal abscesses containing very high amounts. Since these dead white blood cells also rot, as the infection progresses and the numbers of dead cells accumulate dramatically, their rotting contributes to the breakdown of soft tissue and the perpetuation of the disease process.

This moist mixture produces inflammatory components, such as leukotrienes, proinflammatory cytokines, and prostaglandins (each associated with inflammation anywhere in the body), as well as the volatile sulfur compounds (VSCs) hydrogen sulfide and methyl mercaptan. These two VSCs are known to activate collagenase,[1] which breaks down collagen (unfortunately, in the sulcus, this collagen happens to be the sulcular wall in the gum tissue). As previously mentioned, hydrogen sulfide and methyl mercaptan are easy to recognize by their smell—rotten eggs and sewer gas, respectively.

The harmful effects of the toxic stew under the gums, which leads to the breakdown of the gum-tissue wall due to collagenase produced by VSC and other toxic substances, in turn allows up to 400 types of microorganisms to spread throughout the body via the circulatory system. These microorganisms create myriad problems, including inflammation, and have been found in blood clots evaluated at autopsy. Perhaps the most serious effect of all is the inflammation-induced elevation of C-reactive protein. As discussed in Chapter 1, this substance is produced by the liver in response to a wide range of chemical and microbiological causes. CRP circulates at low levels in healthy individuals, but rises considerably in response to infection, inflammation, and injury, and gum disease is associated with all three of these stimuli. If you remember some of Bif's problems, his CRP levels would probably be off the chart. A 1999 article in *Diabetes Care*[2] described a study of 16,573 people in which about "90 percent of apparently healthy individuals have C-reactive protein levels (less than) 3 mg/L and 99 percent have (less than) 10 mg/L," so we can assume that the lower the reading, the better. Gum disease, as we said, can elevate CRP levels to more than 1,000 times the normal healthy upper limit, and I have no doubt the CRP healthy upper limit is being reconsidered as the knowledge of its severe health consequences is becoming better known. CRP levels are directly related to circulating levels of inflammation-inducing blood elements. CRP has been responsible for causing clotting anywhere in the body, including the brain, heart, legs, and lungs.

Collectively, odors, circulating microorganisms, and elevated CRP can exact a terrible toll on a person's health. In the Physicians Health Study[3] that followed a broad range of lower-risk males, it was found that those with the highest CRP levels had triple the risk of a heart attack, as well as double the chances of having a stroke. So to be on the safe side, it is well to reduce all factors that can elevate CRP.

It is "estimated that more than 100,000,000 American adults have moderate to severe periodontal disease, not counting gingivitis or early stage periodontal disease,"[4] so it doesn't take too much guesswork to figure out what might be elevating CRP in much of the United States population. Even worse, the letter (in *Dental Economics,* August 2002) containing the statistics quoted above stated that only 3 percent of the population receives conventional dental treatment in a given year. That means about 97 percent of the population is either receiving "unconventional treatment," or, more likely, no treatment at all. I would agree with that.

You have already read about the stew that builds up in the sulcus and its role in initiating inflammation, so one of the keys to keeping CRP at the lowest levels possible is to control what goes on in the sulcus. In some people, this stew buildup can be negligible and requires only minimal effort to control. These fortunate individuals manifest little or no evidence of disease, yet others can find it very challenging to maintain the cleanliness of the sulcus—and, to repeat, one of the keys to controlling periodontal disease is to keep the sulcus clean. But what percentage of the population even thinks about keeping the sulcus clean on a regular basis?

What makes home-care efforts so vexing for the dentist or hygienist, and so frustrating for their patients who find out their efforts aren't working, is that many people think that state-of-the-art home care is basically just brushing well two or three times a day, and flossing at least once a day. Most people now know to brush and floss after every meal, three times a day, and to floss thoroughly at least once a day, probably because this message has been drummed into their heads over the years in toothpaste or mouthwash advertisements that induce them to buy and use certain products. Unfortunately, the public has been grievously misinformed about brushing, flossing, and using some advertised product; they all still fall short of what's required for genuinely effective oral (systemic) health maintenance, by far, even though together they make up the current standard for oral care.

Let's begin with the shortcomings of brushing. The problem is, although brushing with a manual toothbrush can be very effective at cleaning the teeth from the point of the gum margin, this tool is incapable of doing much to clean down to any significant depth below the gum margins, and certainly not down to the probing depths most people have around their teeth, where the toxic stew resides.

Compounding the frequently ineffectual home-care regimen is the notion that flossing somehow cleans under the gums. It does, but only so far as the soft tissue on the tongue side and cheek side of the tooth will let it. The depth below this level is where most of the disease occurs (gingivitis excepted). While flossing has definite benefits for many who perform this important task, it has been said that only 2 percent of the population flosses every day. Even doubling that to 4 percent still leaves 96 percent of the public not flossing even once a day. And those who *do* floss can't clean the stew out from under the gums. In fact, although flossing does move the plaque and food debris that builds up between the teeth, and does dislodge some of it so it can be cleansed out of the mouth, the balance of the debris is forced into the sulcus.

The pitfalls of home care can be made even worse if you use a toothpaste or mouthwash containing ingredients that carry warnings to "seek professional help or contact a poison control center immediately," and are known to cause harm. And these are products that are supposed to help us get healthy? As mentioned in Chapter 5, my professional advice is to stay away from them. Products containing ingredients that can kill people, induce oral cancer, cause allergic reactions, burning, itching, redness, and soft-tissue sloughing, and degrade tooth-colored fillings and cosmetic dental bonding agents are *not* improving the health of the user. People with gum disease already have enough problems without adding toxic products to their oral health program.

The federal government has compiled much of this disturbing information (oral cancer statistics, alcoholic-mouthwash-ingestion deaths, and so on) and it is available to anyone who is interested in seeing it.[5] Universities and independent research labs have done valuable work to determine other harmful effects of oral health products. ADA-approved or not, if a person is interested in his or her health, these products need to stay undisturbed in their respective tubes and bottles, as colorful displays on the store shelf where they can't possibly do any harm. As far as

I am concerned, oral health can best be accomplished by exclusively using healthy products and techniques.

I would like to make it clear, just for the record, that I am all for brushing and flossing. Both of these activities are fundamental oral health procedures, and both offer benefits if they are done frequently (brushing and flossing have to be done often enough to keep plaque, and other debris removed by these activities, at sufficiently minimal levels to ensure that the gum tissue remains healthy). I especially want a patient's brushing and flossing efforts to be effective and non-injurious, but unfortunately I often see just the opposite. It is extremely common for dentists to see toothbrush abrasion from improper brushing, or the effects of the wrong kind of brush. As I said earlier, hard and medium brushes should only be used for cleaning small motor parts and boots, not teeth. As far as flossing is concerned, gingival clefts (cuts) are also quite common when this procedure is done improperly, and the daily inflammatory injury to the gums not only allows microorganisms into the body but also causes gum and bone recession, even occasional tooth loss. (For some reason, I've seen moderate to severe flossing damage almost exclusively in women, some of it requiring surgery to repair the damage.) These are very poor rewards for such vigorous efforts intended only to improve health. Brushing and flossing *can* both be performed effectively, and without injury, which I will cover in Chapter 7.

I hope the information here and in the previous chapters has convinced you that your oral and systemic health can largely depend on how clean you keep your mouth—and that brushing and flossing can't do it alone. Chapter 7 will outline much of the specific information that has proven beneficial, even lifesaving, in helping my patients recover from both oral and systemic disease. I said it before, but it bears repeating, that the mouth is intimately connected to the whole body, and I hope you can sense that we are entering a new era in which periodontal disease is viewed as a major cause of systemic disease, and gum disease and its inflammatory consequences is understood to cause even death in extreme cases.

The public's perception of periodontal disease and its consequences is, unfortunately, still not yet in tune with the health consequences associated with what is, in fact, a systemic infection. Until those perceptions change on a widespread basis within the medical and dental professions, as well as in the public domain, we will continue to lose the battle. However, perceptions and concepts can occasionally change almost overnight, and I am encouraged that the public and the health professions may soon start viewing periodontal disease and its potentially lethal toll in a totally new light. Only then will any meaningful improvement occur. I don't know if a person's cause of death will ever be listed as gum disease, since it was perhaps a heart attack or a stroke that ultimately caused the death, but I do know that it would certainly help elevate the public's awareness of how serious this health problem is.

7

Winning the Oral Health Game

The information in this chapter is the same information I give to my patients. It is designed to assist you in taking charge of your own oral health, thereby improving it and your systemic health. Because systemic health and oral health are inseparable, I will refer to both as, simply, "health" from here on out. Thanks to my patients, I've had the opportunity to see for myself how effective home-care strategies can work to improve health. I've also seen the damage done to mouths and teeth by the products and devices commonly available today, which even when used *as directed* can inflict sometimes irreparable damage.

As a reminder, I would encourage you to select a dentist and hygienist you trust for her or his assistance in diagnosing your current health status, as well as in helping you monitor your home-care efforts and oral health status. Having a competent and caring dentist and hygienist is essential to your long-term health goals, and your best chance of finding either is probably through word of mouth.

Keep in mind, the mouth is either healthy, or it isn't, and the best evidence that a home-care program is working is a healthy mouth and gums, with no evidence of disease upon probing. If current statistics are accurate, perhaps 5 to 25 percent of the adult population would have no evidence of periodontal disease, as determined by a *complete and thorough periodontal examination* (I estimate that only 2 out of 100 adults will have totally healthy periodontal tissues). So that leaves the majority with less than excellent health and a condition that will not spontaneously reverse itself.

If you are about to be treated for periodontal disease, I recommend that you get a high-sensitivity CRP test before you get too far into professional therapy. It will be a diagnostic baseline marker indicative of the total burden that inflammation is placing on your body. Since the periodontal therapy itself, your home-care efforts, and the top ten nutrients for a healthy mouth, covered in Chapter 8, can all be very effective in reversing CRP levels, be sure you get this test done. (Blood sugar, HDL, LDL, and total cholesterol would be other important baseline tests to have done.) Once you establish a baseline, you can take another CRP test following your therapy to measure the expected success of your efforts to reduce, or even eliminate, disease.

Assuming that action is required if there is periodontal disease, we'll leave the treatment to your dentist and dental hygienist, and take a look at the mundane, but fundamentally important, concept of toothbrushing.

TOOTHBRUSHING AND TOOTHBRUSHES

A toothbrush is merely a device intended to physically clean all the accessible plaque off the teeth and gums that the brush comes in contact with during normal use. Although no manual toothbrush can clean the contacts between the teeth, or effectively go to any meaningful depth in the sulcus where the toxic stew may be, selecting the proper toothbrush is still critical. A manual brush should always be soft, *never* hard or medium, as they can cause severe damage to the teeth over time. They can also cause immediate damage to the delicate soft tissues surrounding the teeth, leading to inflammation and a portal of entry for microorganisms. (Oral surgeons and periodontists are kept continually busy extracting teeth and doing gum surgery to repair the damage done by hard and medium brushes, and I hope you can avoid this.) In addition to never using a hard or medium brush, you should apply only gentle, light pressure when you brush with the recommended soft one, making sure as you brush that no accessible areas are missed. Areas that are consistently overlooked often end up with disease, so take care to be thorough.

As an aside, it is frequently more difficult to perform either tooth extractions or root canals on teeth that have been cut in half by toothbrush abrasion. This is because the teeth can be weaker and easier to break, or the canals have calcified due to persistent stimulation of the

AN IMPORTANT DISTINCTION

To make any discussion of toothbrushes or toothbrushing meaningful, it is well to elaborate upon a critical distinction that my dentist, Dr. Jose M. Gonzalez, Jr., of Laredo, Texas, eloquently brought to my attention several years ago. Dr. Gonzalez told me that he explains the difference between brushing the teeth and cleaning the mouth to his patients by asking them to imagine going to the bathroom and telling themselves they need to brush their teeth. Once this activity is performed, he asks, what is the result? Only brushed teeth. Now, he says, imagine the difference if these same patients are told to go clean their mouths. Does brushing the teeth clean the mouth? Not even close, he says, pointing out that there is a monumental difference between brushing the teeth and cleaning the mouth, and that far more than brushing and flossing is required to accomplish the latter.

Winning the oral health game requires a clean mouth, and brushing is only one essential step in this process. Please keep this important distinction in mind as you read this chapter's discussions of the toothbrushing aspect of safely and effectively cleaning your mouth. A clean mouth requires clean teeth, sulci, tongue, hard and soft palate, and other oral soft tissues, which are more readily achievable when you use the correct products, devices, and techniques.

A super-clean mouth can be attained by conscientiously using the right mouth-cleaning items in the right way.

tooth root, making it virtually impossible to clean out the canal and save the tooth. Additionally, crowns (or caps) on teeth affected by toothbrush abrasion can end up looking too long when the crown has to cover all the exposed root that was once covered by gum tissue. Sometimes cosmetic dental surgery is required to cover the exposed root structure before aesthetic crowns or other cosmetic procedures can be accomplished.

If the right technique is used, soft brushes can easily remove plaque, but no brush can remove hard deposits or stains safely, without damage, and it is too risky to even try doing it by yourself. This is a job for your dentist or hygienist because they are trained and equipped to do it the right way, without damaging your teeth or gum tissue.

Brushing safely and effectively isn't difficult to do, and assuming you have chosen a manual (non-powered) brush, please be certain that the brush is soft, with rounded bristle ends that are capable of cleaning not only above the gum line, but a little bit below it as well. In order to do the job thoroughly, proper brushing involves using a system as well as a technique, so I'll tell you what I always instruct my patients to do. Begin toothbrushing on the cheek sides of the upper right back teeth, by placing the brush at a 45-degree angle to the gum line (see Figure 7.1) and gently brushing in a small back-and-forth motion, two to three teeth at a time, for approximately ten brushing strokes per area. Once this area has been brushed, move toward the front to the next two to three teeth. Continue the process of gently brushing the gum-tooth margin in small, gentle, back-and-forth strokes for at least ten brushing repetitions, or until the area feels adequately cleansed. Then, making sure to keep the bristles angled into the sulcus at approximately a 45-degree angle, continue brushing around the arch two to three teeth at a time until the entire outer surfaces of all the upper teeth have been brushed.

Continue the same process, brushing the tongue side of all the upper teeth systematically, two to three teeth at a time, with the brush angled into the sulcus, until the inner surfaces of all the upper teeth have been brushed. Brushing the inner surfaces of the upper front and lower front teeth is sometimes accomplished more easily if the brush is used vertically and gently moved left and right for ten repetitions, massaging the gum as you go. It's easy to feel the progress of the toothbrush around the arch of the mouth, and being aware of how the brushing feels is important in order to make sure you miss nothing as you proceed.

Brushing the lower teeth is almost the same as brushing the upper teeth except that the bristles are now angled downward at approximately a 45-degree angle in order to help cleanse the lower gum margins effectively. It is important to start on the outside surfaces of the back teeth, either right or left side, and brush two to three teeth at a time, for about ten back-and-forth repetitions before moving on to the next teeth. When all the outside surfaces of the lower teeth have been brushed, the lingual (inside) surfaces are next to be systematically brushed until they have all been cleansed.

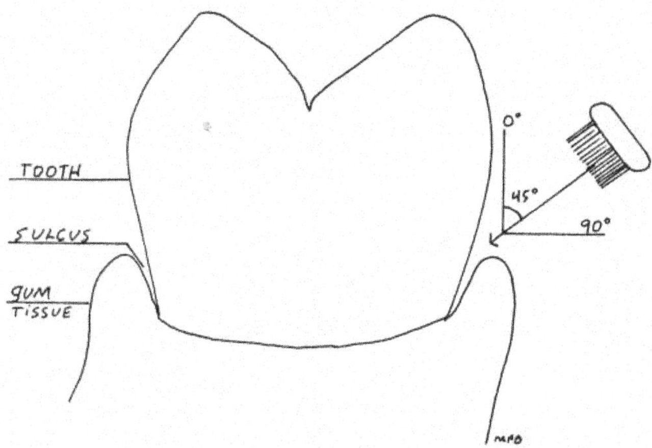

Figure 7.1. Angle your toothbrush into the gum/tooth margin at approximately 45 degrees to facilitate cleaning the sulcus more effectively, and brush gently with a back-and-forth motion.

Are we done brushing at this point? Not quite. It is important to brush the biting surfaces of all the teeth, especially the back ones with the deep grooves, which can trap plaque that can, in turn, cause tooth decay (cavities), odor, and more gum disease. Now are we done brushing?

We're almost done. To finish, use a sideways motion to brush the gum margins at the back of your last teeth on the upper and lower arches, left and right. This step is best done when transitioning from brushing the outside surfaces of the teeth to brushing the inside surfaces, as you turn the corner around the last tooth and start brushing back in the other direction.

What type of brush does the best job? My personal manual toothbrush, the Radius, is an odd-looking but exceedingly effective toothbrush. Being right-handed or left-handed *does* matter here since this particular Radius toothbrush (Radius has normal brushes as well) isn't designed to be used alternatively by either hand. It has to be bought for one or the other because it has a thumb-rest indentation built into the handle of the brush that automatically angles the bristles correctly when brushing at the gum-tooth margins. If you put the brush in the wrong hand, it simply doesn't fit.

The oval-shaped head of the brush is large enough to brush at least two to three teeth at one time, and the outside surfaces of the top and bottom teeth can be brushed at the same time if the upper and lower teeth are touching, or at least close together. I still brush using the system I've described above, but since the brush is so big, and it is angled scientifically to do the job with simple back-and-forth movements, this specific model of the Radius makes brushing effective, efficient, and quick when used properly. But any soft manual brush you choose, and use according to the above instructions, will do a good job of helping you begin the process of cleaning your mouth.

Surprisingly, though, the best toothbrush available isn't even a manual toothbrush; it's an electric one. Studies have shown that the best results can be achieved with these powered toothbrushes, some of which are even capable of loosening debris from the sulcus itself. There are a number of electric brushes available, but the one I presently use, as well as recommend to patients, is a sonic type called the Sonicare. It's easy to use, cleans under the gums to some degree and, at approximately 31,000 brush strokes per minute for a couple of minutes, it gives you an exceptional cleaning with almost no chance of injury to your teeth or gum tissue (assuming you use it properly).

If you wear orthodontic brackets and wires, however, you will often do better with a small rotary electric brush. So, among the many good powered brushes available, find one that you like, and use it according to instructions. Regardless of which powered toothbrush you choose, its cost will ultimately be far less than that of repairing the damage done by a hard or medium brush over a long period of time. Seen in this light, an electric toothbrush is a bargain, and when used properly, it can be exceptionally helpful in keeping the teeth and gums plaque-free. Effective plaque control is fundamental to an effective home-care program, and although it is only one step involved in cleaning the mouth, it is an important one because your health hinges on it. So don't be haphazard about this home-health activity. Brush gently, and brush well.

How often should you brush? It all depends on the individual, but two to three times daily suffices for most people. Right after meals and before bed are the best times to brush. If you find yourself brushing more than three times a day, it is probably too much, and perhaps the other mouth-cleaning activities in this chapter will deliver the feeling you are searching for. Let's go on and find out more about how to win the oral health game.

FLOSSING

Flossing delivers several important health-maintenance benefits. Since microorganisms, both living and dead, build up between the contacts where the teeth touch each other, flossing is important for reducing the possibility and incidence of cavities between the teeth ("interproximal decay" in dentistry terms). Microorganisms at the contacts can process the foods we eat, such as carbohydrates and starches, and in this processing can produce acids that dissolve enamel. So for those who are susceptible to these types of cavities, flossing is exceedingly important in helping to keep decay between the teeth under control. Additionally, for those who have had their fillings, or other types of dental restorations on tooth structure, lost to decay between the teeth, it is imperative to effectively and frequently cleanse the surfaces between the teeth to reduce the incidence of new decay in these areas.

Because microorganisms are so abundant under the gums and are so intermingled with sloughed-off epithelial cells from the gum-tissue wall of the sulcus, it is important to do what we can to keep this toxic mixture to a minimum, consequently reducing the chances of early-stage gum infections (gingivitis) or the more advanced stages of infection and destruction associated with periodontal disease. Properly done, flossing can be very effective at dislodging accumulated plaque and cellular debris from the sulcular spaces between the teeth, allowing this plaque to be ultimately removed from the mouth, usually by expectoration (spitting it out).

How do we floss properly? The first step, in my opinion, is to choose a brand and type of floss that works for you, one you can, and will, use. There is a confusing array of flosses available: waxed and unwaxed, dental tape (wider than floss and easier on the fingers for those with tight contacts), flavored flosses, and even floss in a handheld device that allows flossing to be done with one hand. Although dentists and hygienists have been known to draw swords over the relative merits of waxed versus unwaxed floss, the best floss is ultimately one that you will use every day. Start trying out various flosses until you find one you like. Whatever self-motivation it takes to include flossing as an everyday component of your oral-cleansing activities, do it. I'm sure I'd approve of your choice.

Besides all the health benefits of flossing, one further motivator could be that flossing makes breath fresher. Fresh breath is difficult to achieve when loads of necrotic, stinking plaque is left under the gums and between the teeth for long periods of time. Since patients with bad breath seldom smell their own halitosis, they may not even be aware their breath is offensive. A simple test to see if you have a problem is simply to floss, then smell the floss. The odor, if present, will become worse as the plaque dries. One thing is for certain, flossing and fresh breath go hand in hand: no one has ever had bad breath worsen by having a cleaner mouth.

If you still need encouragement to floss daily, consider this: the words *floss* and *heart* both have five letters. While this observation may seem silly, flossing can keep the inflammation caused by gum disease at lower, safer levels. So if you aren't flossing for fresh breath and healthier gum tissue, or working to keep your cavities and the decay between your teeth under control, then floss for better heart health.

How do you go about flossing safely, easily, and effectively? You've chosen your floss already, so the following is the same information I pass on to my patients. Hopefully it will work for you. But first, please review Figures 7.2 and 7.3; these are diagrams that I draw for my patients. They will help you understand what floss can, and cannot, accomplish.

I instruct my patients to take an eighteen-inch section of floss and wind it equally around the middle fingers of each hand until the index fingers or the thumbs on each hand are close enough to touch. This allows the floss to be directed and controlled, by using both thumbs to direct the floss if flossing the upper teeth, or by using the index fingers when flossing the lower teeth (making sure to use only gentle motions throughout the flossing).

With one to two inches of floss in between, start by flossing the front of the last tooth on the upper right. By using a system, you won't miss anything, and by starting in the same place every time you floss, your flossing will become a habit. Keep the floss taut with your fingers, and with your thumbs, direct it between your upper teeth, then guide it through the contact and scrub the front of the last tooth, up and down, with just a slight amount of rocking motion, until you feel that the surface of the tooth is clean. You have just flossed the front of the tooth and

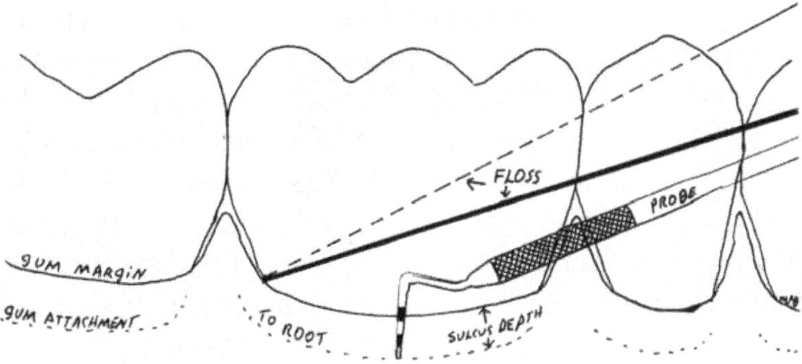

Figure 7.2. Flossing is an excellent way to clean between the teeth and partially into the sulcus at the fronts and backs of the teeth.

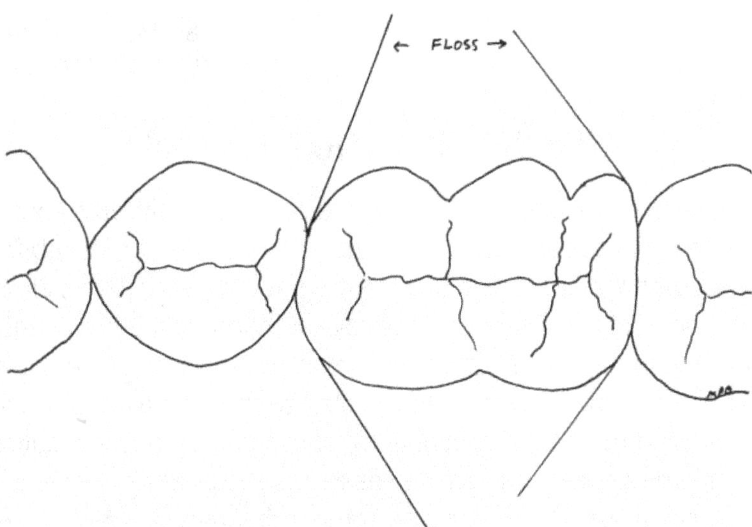

Figure 7.3. The view of the top of the teeth in Figure 7.3 demonstrates that, although flossing cannot cleanse the sulcus on either the cheek sides or the tongue sides of the teeth, it is very effective at cleaning the tooth-to-tooth contacts and dislodging plaque and food debris from between the teeth.

cleansed the part of the sulcus at that tooth. The next step is to lift the floss over the gum tissue between the two teeth and floss the back of the next tooth, the one directly in front of the first one you flossed. Remove the floss from between the teeth and insert it into the next contact forward. Floss the front of one tooth and the back of the next tooth and move on to the next contact. Please remember you are not just cleaning the front of one tooth, but you are also cleaning the back of the next one, as well as cleaning a bit of the sulcular debris from both sides of the gum tissue in between the teeth (the interdental papillae).

Then, move on to the lower teeth, again systematically flossing to ensure that no surfaces will be missed. You can floss effectively between the lower teeth by keeping the floss taut and directing it between the teeth using your index fingers. If the floss tears or frays from the effects of really tight contacts, rough fillings, or sharp edges between the teeth, just release one wind of floss from one middle finger and take up the slack by winding it onto the other middle finger.

Assuming you have a full complement of teeth, you can do a very effective job of flossing in about a minute and a half, so the potential reward in improved health will be a good enough reason to include flossing as an important part of your daily health-maintenance regimen.

PREVENTING TOOTH DECAY

Since effective brushing and flossing are absolutely critical in controlling dental decay in susceptible individuals, I want to detour for a brief discussion about the cause and prevention of tooth decay. Three elements need to be in place before tooth decay can happen: the microorganism responsible for decay (*Streptococcus mutans*) must be present, a sugar or carbohydrate for *S. mutans* to metabolize must be available, and the tooth or teeth must be susceptible to, or capable of, decay. Additionally, there are three cavity-preventing measures those of us susceptible to tooth decay must take in order to combat this decay: we must control plaque, reduce carbohydrates (sugars) in our diet, and make our teeth more resistant to decay.

The tooth decay equation is pretty simple: bugs plus sugar equals acid production. These acids can dissolve enamel as well as tooth-root structure and result in a cavity (technically, a carious lesion). Although tooth decay is a fact of life for almost everyone, there are some lucky people who simply do not experience it because their teeth are resistant to the acids the *S. mutans* bacterium produces in its processing of sugar or other carbohydrates.

Eliminating, or at least drastically reducing, tooth decay is certainly doable, but it takes a little effort. Proper brushing and flossing are of paramount importance in eliminating tooth decay in the caries-susceptible individual because, without excellent control of plaque (the sticky stuff containing cavity-causing microorganisms, including *S. mutans*), cavities can develop in the grooves (pits and fissures) of the teeth, in between the teeth, on the sides of the teeth at the gum margins, and on the roots of the teeth. Tooth decay at the margins (edges) of fillings, crowns, or bridges distresses dentists and patients alike, since much of this restorative work was done to repair damage caused by previous decay, and new decay around existing dental work does not usually get restored properly with a patchwork approach. Once the dentist has done his or her best to restore a tooth, this work needs to be well maintained by the patient, and this book contains information that will help anyone who is serious about doing so.

Brushing and flossing are critical in controlling the plaque that can lead to decay, but further reduction of microorganisms is necessary for a healthy mouth. This can be achieved by tongue scraping (the top of most peoples' tongues harbor untold trillions of microorganisms and much odorous material), and irrigation to reduce the number of microorganisms under the gum margins. The use of the toothpastes I recommend in the next section can make a very significant difference in reducing microorganisms, and the use of either the BGSE Mint Mouthwash Treatment, or the Oxyfresh Fresh Mint Mouthrinse with Zinc after brushing, flossing, and tongue scraping can offer significant benefits as well. Irrigation is fully covered later in this chapter, but I can recommend either mouthwash mentioned above for use in a home-based hydromagnetic irrigator to flush plaque out from under the gum margins, as well as out from between the teeth. This additional reduction in decay-causing plaque not only has oral health benefits but can also help lower dental costs.

An obvious way to cut down on dental decay is to reduce or even eliminate sugary drinks from the diet. Great plaque control is an excellent way to keep cavity-causing organisms at lower levels in the mouth, but even great plaque control is no match for the acids produced when six to twelve sugar-containing soft drinks are consumed every day; this much sugar coating the teeth supports the astronomically fast growth of the cavity-causing organism and its acids. Coffee or tea sweetened with sugar will create never-ending cavities in anyone prone to decay, as I learned from personal experience years ago, despite exceptional plaque-control efforts with brushing and flossing. The use of nonsugar sweeteners is recommended for those susceptible to tooth decay; the one I recommend (and use) is Splenda. It's safe and won't cause tooth decay.

Another excellent way to deal with dental decay is to drink several cups of green tea a day. Why is green tea so great for reducing dental decay? One study showed that green tea actually inhibits the growth of plaque caused by the *S. mutans* bacteria,[1] while another study showed "that green tea catechins actually destroyed these bacteria at concentrations lower than those found in only one cup of tea."[2] Other studies report that green tea strongly inhibits bacteria after only five to ten minutes of exposure to the tea.[3] And yet another study reported that green tea extract was more effective than fluoride compounds in preventing dental caries.[4]

To summarize, consuming three or four cups of green tea daily for dental reasons is a great idea because it inhibits the growth of plaque caused by *S. mutans,* destroys the biofilm that coats teeth and the rest of the mouth (thus helping to clean the mouth), and, because of the fluoride content in green tea, actually makes the teeth more resistant to acids produced by *S. mutans.* Fluoride in its many dental formulations is actually the third method that has been utilized to reduce susceptibility to tooth decay (caries) in cavity-prone individuals. I get mine from green tea and recommend the same to my patients. Please note that when consuming green tea for its cavity-reducing benefits, it is best to swish each mouthful of green tea vigorously to cleanse the mouth before swallowing the tea. In other words, don't just drink the tea as you normally would, since the cleansing action and the *S. mutans* inhibition are improved by having the tea in contact with the mouth and teeth for longer periods of time.

Finally, my advice on the use of green tea is to find one you like, and have it readily available at work and at home so you can drink it on a regular basis. Green tea has benefits that go well beyond reducing cavities, and you can take advantage of them all if you will incorporate drinking several cups into your normal daily routine. Green tea is so important that I give my patients samples as well as instructions for its use. (For additional information on green tea, see Chapter 8.)

A final note on the dental decay issue: make certain that you have regular dental checkups. Your dentist is there to help you be healthy, and regular dental visits afford the greatest possibility of keeping dental problems at a minimum.

TOOTHPASTES AND MOUTHWASHES

You've already read about toxic toothpastes and scary mouthwashes, so you realize we can't win the oral health game if we use products that cause problems, some quite serious. That being said, most people give little thought to the toothpaste or mouthwash they use, other than what they want it to do for them. Toothpastes in particular are promoted as offering any number of benefits that the consumer might consider a good reason to buy the product. The more common advertisements promote toothpastes that whiten teeth; toothpastes than desensitize teeth; toothpastes that freshen breath; toothpastes that kill germs; toothpastes that control tartar; toothpastes that fight plaque; toothpastes that offer cavity protection; toothpastes that fight cavities; and the most inclusive of all, a toothpaste that helps prevent cavities, fights bad breath and gingivitis, helps prevent plaque, and fights tartar as well. The truth is, this last kind of toothpaste might actually do some of what is promised because one of its ingredients is triclosan, a pesticide registered with the Environmental Protection Agency (EPA). It helps us *exterminate* plaque.

There is plenty of choice in considering which toothpaste to buy, but the choices narrow considerably if you choose a toothpaste that is able to deliver many of the oral health benefits we all require, while also being reasonably safe to use. Obviously, most toothpastes would not carry warnings to consult a physician, or contact a poison control center immediately if the product is swallowed, if they were not required to do so. Another perplexing thought is, why is it safe to use a product at thirteen years of age when it carries warnings for those under age twelve? The fluoride content desired for cavity prevention can discolor, or even destroy, enamel if too much fluoride is ingested, so it is especially important to avoid too much fluoride until at least age twelve, the age by which all the enamel of all the teeth (wisdom teeth excepted) has been formed. Monitoring whether a child has swallowed toothpaste or not can be very difficult for parents, dentists, or hygienists to manage. (Fluoridated toothpaste isn't the only hazard to healthy teeth, since many areas of the country have very high levels of fluoride in their water supplies; infants as well as children up to age twelve should drink purified water instead, to avoid receiving too much fluoride that can lead to severe dental defects.)

As I advised in Chapter 5, it would be well to take another look at what you use in your oral health home-care program. Toothpastes and mouthwashes need to be effective *and* safe, and although a few toothpastes and mouthwashes available do come close to filling that bill, most don't come close enough. While they may contain mostly natural ingredients that do benefit the user, the manufacturer will then include sodium lauryl sulfate (SLS) so the product will foam. SLS doesn't belong in oral health products because it is itself a major cause of health problems.

A recent article in the peer-reviewed journal of the Academy of General Dentistry[5] reported on case studies in which SLS was associated with a rather long list of oral mucosal problems. Among the lesions reported were "mucosal desquamation; mucosal irritation; epithelial sloughing; contact cheilitis; recurrent aphthous ulcers (three reports of RAU); painful desquamation; and burning sensation." Read your toothpaste labels, and if your product contains SLS or other harmful ingredients (see Chapter 5 for a list), you will quickly absorb these ingredients into your oral soft tissues, so it would be best not to use it.

Chlorhexidine, a prescription mouthwash high in alcohol that is commonly prescribed to combat gum disease, was also referred to in the report outlining the problems associated with SLS. One case noted "fixed drug eruption," while the other said there was "acute swelling/ulceration of lips." It is unfortunate that commercial toothpastes and mouthwashes continue to be a potentially constant source of oral health problems, but an informed consumer who has made the decision to use only healthful products can opt out of the risk merely by reading the labels and choosing not to use dangerous products.

What are toothpastes and mouthwashes supposed to do? The ideal toothpaste would facilitate cleaning the teeth when brushing, as well as provide cavity protection and have an antimicrobial (acting against bacteria, fungi, spores, viruses, and yeast) effect on those organisms remaining in the mouth. Breath-freshening benefits and desensitizing effects would be helpful. Any ingredients that facilitate healing would also be very beneficial inclusions, since the ailing oral soft tissues could absorb them. The product would be harmless both to existing dental work and to the patient, with a very low incidence of sensitivity to any of the ingredients (I've had patients who would break out in a rash when something as harmless as water got on their skin, so no product is ever suitable for every user). There may be other benefits a particular user would like their ideal toothpaste to have, but few brands of toothpaste available at the present time can honestly be called safe *and* effective. At least there *are* a few, and as I mentioned in Chapter 5, I personally use and recommend a product containing grapefruit seed extract since it is exceedingly effective as a toothpaste, is totally safe, and has all-natural organic ingredients, which benefit us most when they are *allowed* to remain in contact with the oral soft tissues rather than get rinsed out immediately after use. Including additional ingredients, such as green tea, methylsulfonylmethane (MSM), several essential oils, and other healthful organic ingredients, the product I like (BGSE Mint Toothpaste) is exceptional.

Since paste is often left in the mouth after brushing, why not take advantage of a good product's potential benefits and floss it under the gum margins and between the teeth instead of rinsing it out? Extracts of green tea, MSM, grapefruit seed extracts, and other antioxidants discussed earlier in connection with toothpaste offer such numerous health benefits that each has been the subject of entire books. Since all these ingredients offer antimicrobial benefits, and some are exceedingly anti-inflammatory and are *required* for healthy gum tissue, I instruct my patients to floss residual toothpaste under the gums. My patients who have done this over the years have almost universally seen better gum-tissue health in the first few weeks of following this procedure with BGSE toothpaste, and their long-term results have been very good to excellent. Additionally, I have never seen a patient of mine using BGSE toothpaste have any sort of soft-tissue reaction such as we commonly see in patients who have used toothpaste containing any of the untouchables discussed in Chapter 5. People who want to win the battle against gum disease have a better chance of success with a regimen such as this. (Please be aware that my clinical observations of the health benefits observed in numerous patients using BGSE toothpaste are mine alone. The manufacturer only claims that the paste "safely cleans and whitens teeth, freshens breath and invigorates clean-feeling gums," and makes *no* therapeutic claims.)

Given that there are few toothpastes available that I would use or recommend other than the preferred one I've mentioned already, choose your toothpaste carefully. I know from experience that patients can be quite fond of a particular brand of toothpaste. If their mouths are healthy, I encourage them to keep doing whatever they've been doing, unless they might want to take a look at something that would be even better. If they are healthy, it's their choice, but if they are not, discussions are in order.

The situation with available mouthwashes is the same as that with the widely available commercial toothpastes. Most mouthwashes are loaded with harmful ingredients. They are meant to cleanse and freshen the mouth, as well as deodorize, but most accomplish these ends with highly flavored, alcohol-based solutions that merely mask one odor by covering it up with a stronger one. Since the breath-freshening effect lasts only a short time, a person with halitosis has to turn frequently to the product, as often as every thirty minutes, which results in a chronic exposure of her or his oral soft tissues to substances that are known to carry health risks. Remember Bif, and the shape he was in? He was swishing with his 60-proof mouthwash every thirty minutes. As with toothpaste, some products are safer than others, the alcohol-free ones being obvious improvements over their alcoholic competitors. When used properly, a safe, effective mouthwash can make a significant difference in mouth cleanliness and fresh breath. Proper use would include using the mouthwash three to four times a day, and rinsing with it vigorously and long enough to give the ingredients time to provide the desired benefits—healthier gums, fresher breath, and a clean-feeling mouth.

Among the very few safe and effective mouthwashes that contain ingredients designed to facilitate oral health are organic products that I use and recommend. BGSE Mint Mouthwash Treatment is one of them. It has a number of safe, effective ingredients, and contains none that should never touch your lips. As previously stated, its antimicrobial effect is based on a bioflavonoid derived from grapefruit seed extract. This ingredient not only has antimicrobial properties, but its bioflavonoids are important in healing because they play a role in the formation of collagen, the connective-tissue building block that is a required component of bone and cartilage, as well as gum tissue, muscles, skin—everything.

The only other mouthwash I strongly recommend is Oxyfresh Fresh Mint Mouthrinse with Zinc, described as a stabilized chlorine dioxide rinse containing zinc acetate. This safe mouthwash is exceedingly effective at cleansing the mouth while eliminating odors.

At the present time, mouthwash is routinely used by those attempting to mask oral malodor or heal sore spots in the mouth, for instance bleeding or sore gums, but few, if any, readily available, off-the-shelf mouthwashes do much to help either situation. Since a safe, effective mouthwash can be highly instrumental in helping its user have a cleaner, healthier, and fresher mouth, I would like to propose that more people think about incorporating the use of a good mouthwash into their daily oral health efforts. The results that you can achieve in just a few weeks of conscientious mouthwash use, with an effective product, will very likely lead you to add this important mouth-cleansing step to your daily program.

Additionally, for those who wear removable dental appliances of any sort, please remember that, because they are in the mouth, they build up microorganisms and odors, and can contribute to increased tooth decay, gum disease, and odor if they are not cleaned daily using the same safe and effective products that are used in the mouth. It makes no sense whatsoever to diligently clean the mouth and then put a contaminated, odorous appliance back into the mouth. Cleansing the mouth means making the dental appliances worn in the mouth as clean as the mouth itself, and using the same safe, effective products to do so.

There are literally hundreds of toothpastes and mouthwashes available, including good ones I may not be aware of, as well as the more prevalent bad ones that need to be left on the shelf. It is very important to read the labels and choose products designed to actually enhance your oral health rather than retard it. As a practicing dentist myself, I can assure you, from observing my patients, that very rapid improvement in oral health can occur when good products replace the bad. Since winning the oral health game requires the use of a safe, effective toothpaste and mouthwash, it is vital to choose your products carefully.

TONGUE SCRAPING

Tongue scraping is a daily health-maintenance procedure that very few people bother with, probably because they don't yet realize they need to keep their tongues clean. However, maintaining fresh breath and healthy gum tissue means you have to remove plaque on a regular basis to keep both your breath and tongue fresh and healthy; food debris, odorous dead bacteria and skin cells, as well as stagnant oral fluids have health and social consequences that are largely avoidable. Nobody wants bad breath or gum disease, and this section will show you how to take better control of both problems through the use of a tongue scraper.

Why should we bother to scrape our tongues? First, it is important to realize that the tongue doesn't have a smooth surface, as most people assume. Rather, it is covered by wormlike projections called filiform papillae that can be long or short, and generally number in the thousands (these are not the taste buds). One way to visualize these filiform papillae is to compare them to a shag rug. The wet, not-very-clean shag is what the upper surface of the tongue is like in the majority of people I've seen over the years. And that's a big problem. The surface area of the tongue gets magnified considerably when you take into account all these projections, and in among these papillae is the same stew that is in the sulcus. But the larger surface area of the tongue may harbor many more microorganisms than all the sulci together might contain; there can literally be trillions of living, dying, rotting, stinking microorganisms on the top of your tongue, which are passively wreaking havoc on your health and social life. Dead skin cells, food debris, and oral fluids are literally saturating the area around the papillae, intermingling with the innumerable microorganisms—and they are most definitely not harmless or unnoticed by others (take bad breath, for example).

Whether the stew is on the tongue or trapped in the sulci makes little difference. It still stinks, still causes soft tissue breakdown, and still creates inflammation, sometimes dramatically. Some patients' tongues will be quite tender, and will bleed when I begin my tongue-scraping efforts—not surprising, considering that the same tissue-destroying enzymes and odors that are under the gums in the sulci are in the stew on the top of the tongue. The tenderness and bleeding usually abate quickly once the tongue gets cleaned daily. And this healing process gets accelerated if effective oral health products and nutritional supplements become part of the regimen.

Tongue-cleaning devices have only appeared in stores and pharmacies in the last few years, brought on by the fresh-breath movement in dentistry that emphasizes tongue scraping as part of the routine needed for nice, fresh breath. A variety of tongue scrapers are available, and what works best for one person might not be suitable for another. You will need to do a little research to find what works best for you. Most scrapers come either as a plastic strip with serrated edges, or as a single-handled metal or plastic device with a scraping edge at one end. Some resemble a rake, others have a loop of metal or plastic that serves as the scraping edge, and all work best when placed firmly at the back of the extended tongue, then are firmly pulled forward along the tongue toward its tip. If you're a beginner, the sheer amount of odorous material you pull forward can be unsettling, but daily efforts will diminish the amounts and help you win this battle.

When scraping the tongue, it is very important to make sure you scrape as far back as possible, since getting rid of microorganisms and odorous debris depends on how effectively this step is performed. The gag reflex can be a problem for some just starting this important health habit, but it is usually overcome quickly and generally ceases to be a problem, especially in anyone determined to have fresh breath. Having a healthy mouth and fresh breath can be a powerful motivator. The tongue-scraping procedure is an important step toward that end, and will add no more than ten or fifteen seconds to your oral health program. (Vigorously swishing with a safe, effective mouthwash after tongue scraping is a particularly effective way to enhance fresh breath, by removing additional microorganisms and neutralizing residual odor.)

How do you know when your tongue is clean? You'll know when you are scraping and no longer getting any odorous residue, and when your tongue is totally pink. A few individuals have short, sparse, or absent filiform papillae on the dorsum (top) of the tongue, and for them, it may not be necessary to cleanse the tongue, as the self-cleansing action of eating and swallowing may be all that's required. Most people, however, will best be served by buying a tongue scraper that meets their needs and implementing tongue scraping as an everyday health-enhancing habit. The difference in mouth cleanliness and freshness will be noticeable very quickly, and if bleeding or tenderness occurs at first, it will generally stop if the tongue is scraped frequently enough to allow healing to progress. Occasionally, someone could have a condition that affects the top of the tongue, such as bacterial or viral lesions, or problems caused by vitamin deficiencies. If scraping causes pain for more than just a few days, seek professional advice. Oral cancer often affects the lateral border of the tongue, so any lesions that don't heal are of particular concern and should be checked out immediately by a dentist or physician.

The concept of cleaning the mouth, as opposed to the current standard of just brushing the teeth, requires that daily tongue scraping be included as an integral component of any effective oral-health, fresh-breath home-care system. Once you have experienced what a really clean mouth feels like, it's unlikely you will accept anything less. Think about it this way: If you have brushed your teeth, but not scraped your tongue, how far do you think the several trillion microorganisms on the tongue have to travel to contaminate the gum tissue and teeth you have just brushed? Not very far.

SULCULAR IRRIGATION

This section discusses one method that will allow you to really begin taking control of cleaning your mouth under the gums where, as you recall, gum disease can establish itself if allowed to do so. This critically important home-care step is accomplished by using the highly effective cleansing ability of a pulsating oral irrigator, which has ionized water jetting through one of a variety of available tips. This cleansing activity offers substantial health benefits by allowing the user to cleanse the sulcus on a daily basis. The same machine can also be used to deliver a number of substances into the sulcus that can kill microorganisms, eliminate odors, or reduce inflammation; it can even bring anti-inflammatory, antioxidant-rich nutrient solutions into the sulcus where any inflamed gum tissue can benefit from them.

In numerous studies, special types of pulsating, hydromagnetic irrigators have been shown to offer benefits, including plaque removal and dissolution of hard deposits, that are simply unachievable without the use of hydromagnetic irrigation. Hydromagnetic irrigators ionize water

(H_2O is a polar molecule capable of being affected by a magnetic field) by forcing the water stream to flow past powerful magnets just moments before this ionized solution is emitted from the irrigation tip. At least two studies have shown that this decidedly low-tech approach is, alternatively, *almost* twice as effective,[6] or *more than* twice as effective[7] in removing plaque as nonmagnetic irrigators.

The effectiveness of moving water to push things in its path forward needs little explanation. Most people have used a stream of water from a hose to clean cracks in driveways or sidewalks, so downsizing this concept to clean the sulcular groove around and between the teeth isn't far-fetched.

The great thing about hydromagnetic irrigators is that they combine the ability of ionization to reduce surface tension with the force of moving water. Let me explain. Many people have played with either horseshoe-shaped or round, coin-shaped magnets and have observed that the magnets either powerfully attract one another, or just as powerfully repel one another. In fact, many of you have probably pushed one magnet across a smooth surface with another magnet, and had fun doing so because it was fascinating to observe that some unseen force was moving another object without actually touching that object. Therefore, as many of you have observed, while magnetism is invisible, by its effects we know it to be a real, and sometimes powerful, force.

Several theories have been postulated on how hydromagnetic irrigators work better than nonmagnetic irrigators, but my explanation to patients begins with a discussion of how the magnets they may have played with displayed attractive or repulsive forces of equal strength. I then transfer that concept down into the sulcus by explaining that calculus (tartar) is nothing more than microorganisms that have been electromagnetically attracted to the tooth root, and have become established there long enough to colonize and eventually mineralize, forming the hard deposits we know as calculus, or tartar. If we are able to disrupt the ability of microorganisms to adhere to the tooth root, we have interrupted the process that allows the buildup of destructive hard deposits, plaque, and their associated toxins, and have ultimately enhanced the health of the sulcus. Obviously, no one has ever seen a pair of magnets occurring naturally under the gums in the sulcus, but I explain to my patients that, according to researchers, the ability of microorganisms to adhere to the tooth root is based on the fact that the microorganisms carry a negative charge and the tooth root carries a positive charge, hence the bugs are attracted to the tooth root. While the technical details of the actual process are well beyond the scope of this book, this simple explanation can arm you with the concept of how a magnetic irrigator can disrupt the game that microorganisms are playing and keep the damage they can do under control.

When it comes to being more in control of your oral health by using the hydromagnetic irrigator—especially when you add any of the recommended substances to the warm tap water in the irrigator's reservoir—you can drastically improve your situation. You can go from a condition that seems almost hopeless to a more positive one because your mouth begins to feel better due to reduced inflammation and soreness. Irrigators can never reverse an irreversible process; for example, it cannot rebuild bone around a tooth that has lost so much the tooth needs to be extracted. But if we are dealing with inflammation and swelling due to plaque buildup and hard deposits, or pocket formation due to attachment loss and a deepening of the sulcus, the proper use of an irrigator with appropriate irrigants in it, and some of the appropriate supplements discussed in Chapter 8, can lead to results that you, your dentist, and your hygienist will appreciate.

Based on scientific studies, it's been obvious for some time that magnetic irrigators are approximately twice as effective at removing plaque as their nonmagnetic counterparts, but it gets even better. One study indicated that just by using plain water in irrigators with a magnetic device, the users were able to reduce their calculus (hard deposit or tartar) volume by 44 percent—as well as reduce its area by 42 percent more than a comparable group of subjects who used the same irrigators with the magnets removed. Remarkably, removing the magnets had the effect of reducing the irrigators' efficiency nearly 100 percent. Remember, we are cleansing the sulcus here; some of the plaque and hard deposits this technology is capable of affecting are in the sulcus, so the user is now capable of doing a much more effective job of cleansing that area than brushing and flossing alone could ever accomplish.

Irrigation has led to a quantum leap in oral health for many of my patients who have adopted it as a home health-maintenance strategy, and in fourteen years of recommending irrigators to patients, not one of them has ever wanted to discontinue using one. Part of the reason may be that they are shown how to use the machines properly in order to address their specific oral health needs, and because they are individually advised on what to put into the water to increase the irrigator's benefit to them. Knowing every aspect of how to use the irrigator is important; when my patients know how, when, and why to use one, they experience some degree of improvement and get results they can appreciate. This, in turn, helps foster greater compliance with their entire recommended home health-maintenance regimen. While individual successes vary, overall success encourages many patients to continue a process they can see is working. We will go into greater detail on the how's and why's of irrigation, which represent a critically important part of regaining and maintaining everyone's oral health (including mine).

Why is irrigation such an important home health-maintenance step? Chapter 3 discussed the sulcus, that space between the tooth and its gum-tissue wall where up to 400 types of microorganisms live, multiply, and die. It also discussed how this space is the natural dumpsite of the skin cells that are constantly sloughing off the sulcular soft-tissue wall, and most people do not need this book to know that food debris ("food impaction" in dental terminology) is regularly introduced into the sulcus during the act of chewing. In short, as ingredients are constantly being added to the stew, the sulcus is continually being contaminated by a variety of organic materials destined to decompose quickly if left in there where warmth, moisture, and proteolytic enzymes exist to speed the decomposition process along. This odorous, stinky concoction in the sulcus, with the sulcus encircling the entire tooth root, plays a major role in the inflammatory process, frequently causing the breakdown of soft tissue and initiating gum disease. The enzymes, toxins, and gases, if left in the sulcus, will ulcerate and break down the protective barrier in susceptible individuals, thus leading to periodontal disease and its systemic consequences. The social impact is prominent as well, since most would agree that it can be very unpleasant to be too close to someone with bad breath.

When you think of all the putrefaction going on in the sulcus, fresh breath and robust oral and systemic health will almost certainly never be accomplished unless the sulcus is cleansed on a frequent enough schedule. How frequently you need to irrigate, and what the best irrigant to use in the water is, is generally determined over the course of a few visits with the dental team responsible for coaching you toward health. Using the same regimen for everybody would likely result in overdoing it for many, and grossly underdoing it for a few, so achieving the desired results from irrigation often takes some fine-tuning. Your dentist and hygienist can help with this, as can the information here.

As I have repeatedly said, infection and inflammation play a big role in the initiation of gum disease. Two pathogenic organisms that exist primarily in the sulcus, *Porphyromonas gingivalis* and *Actinobacillus actinomycetemcomitans,*[8] are known to cause the inflammatory response seen in periodontal disease. The subject of additional risk factors in periodontal disease is of increasing interest, with gender (males are more susceptible), smoking habits, pre-existing conditions, heredity, and age being considered.[9] For the purposes of this section, however, it's bad enough that the sulcus is the space where just about everything that gets into it goes on to decompose, regardless of other factors. The good news is that, unless you have probing depths greater than 4 mm, it's actually quite easy to cleanse the sulcus through the proper use of a hydromagnetic irrigator (see Figure 7.4). Even for pocket or sulcus depths greater than 4 mm, it is still easy to cleanse the sulcus by using special tips that will allow you to irrigate daily to a depth of at least 6 mm or more (see Figure 7.5).

Although irrigation is frequently performed as a part of periodontal cleanings in-office, the dental profession hasn't yet placed much emphasis on irrigation at home. If you've had this procedure done, you know how fresh and clean your mouth feels. Unfortunately, unless you perform the same service for yourself every day, it won't stay fresh for long. The bacteria, dead skin cells, and food debris reappear (and the microorganisms recolonize) very quickly, building up to levels that probably caused the bleeding gums initially, as well as reinitiating the disease process that caused the periodontal pockets (and other indications of gum disease—usually bleeding and loose teeth, pus, redness, or swelling) many sought dental care for in the first place. Once in-office therapy has been done, whether it was scaling and root planing or even periodontal surgery, no rational individual would want to allow the same pathological conditions to reestablish themselves, thus beginning the whole destructive process over again, would they? Of course not. So, for

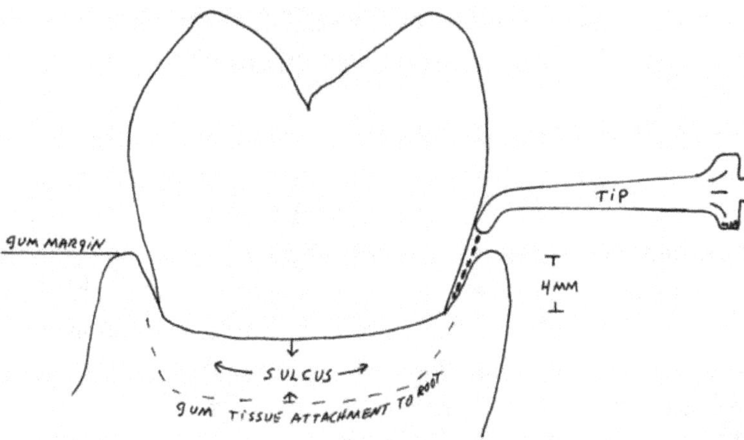

Figure 7.4. The irrigator tip directs a pulsating jet of ionized water up to 4 mm into the sulcus, which flushes out dead microorganisms, cellular debris, toxins, odors, and food particles.

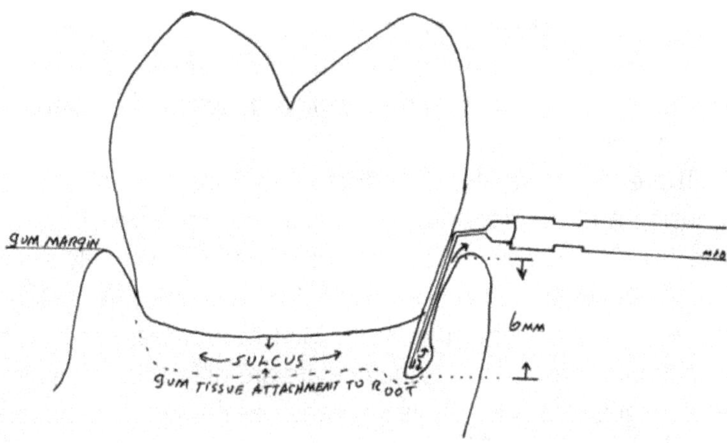

Figure 7.5. Periodontal pockets up to 6 mm deep can be thoroughly cleansed and medicated on a daily basis using a thin side-port cannula with either the Hydrofloss or OxyCare 3000 set at their lowest flow-rate setting.

maximum health benefits, irrigation is best performed every single day, and for some people (including the author), twice a day, morning and evening.

When it comes to buying a hydromagnetic irrigator, it's not like going to Baskin-Robbins where you have thirty-one flavors to choose from. At the hydromagnetic irrigator store, there are currently only two types to choose from. Since I've used both of them and have recommended hundreds of each to my patients, the consistent results that both units have shown indicate we are not missing out on anything by having a limited selection.

The pioneer in hydromagnetics is Hydrofloss, and they make an easy-to-use unit that comes with four different-colored tips so several users can have their own tip while sharing the same irrigator. Hydrofloss users experience a very gentle, but effective, pulsating water stream from the unit. Hydrofloss also has special attachments to allow irrigation to sulcular depths greater than 4 mm, for those who need them. The warranty on the machine together with the good service makes the Hydrofloss highly recommendable for most of my adult patients.

The other hydromagnetic irrigator currently available, OxyCare 3000, is also a fine machine. Available from Oxyfresh, it is a very reliable unit and has a forceful stream of pulsating water when set at its maximum flow rate. Other than that, this machine is quite similar to the Hydrofloss. The OxyCare 3000 also comes with four tips allowing multiple users for the same machine. I make no distinction between their relative effectiveness because I have seen excellent results in hundreds of patients using either machine.

There are several very effective options to really maximize the cleansing and deodorizing effects of either the Hydrofloss or the OxyCare 3000. The two I recommend to patients virtually every day are the mouthwashes I discussed earlier in this chapter. While the chemistry and technology behind the BGSE Mint Mouthwash Treatment and the Oxyfresh Mouthrinse with Zinc Acetate are different, using either in your hydromagnetic irrigator offers so many health-improving possibilities that it would be an oversight not to recommend them. The Oxyfresh product enhances the removal of plaque from the mouth when it is swished vigorously for sixty seconds using one ounce of mouthwash to fifteen ounces of warm water in the irrigator, and its cleansing and deodorizing effect in the sulcus may last for hours. Neither the stabilized chlorine dioxide nor the zinc acetate in this product will ever be a microorganism's best friend, and this product's use in either irrigator has helped my patients reduce inflammation and achieve nearly miraculous results in oral cleanliness. (Note that Oxyfresh makes no therapeutic claims for any of its products, and these observations are mine alone.)

For equally astonishing results derived from a natural combination of organic products, the BGSE Mint Mouthwash Treatment combines the beneficial effects of grapefruit seed extract and hesperidin (both bioflavonoids) with other soothing ingredients, including aloe vera gel and essential oils from anise, menthol, peppermint, spearmint, and wintergreen. The manufacturer, FreeLife International, only claims that this product invigorates and cleanses the gums, and helps you experience long-lasting fresh breath, but my familiarity with what the experts have written about these ingredients, as well as my own personal and clinical observation, leads me to suggest putting two or three capfuls of this mouthwash in your irrigator and trying it out for a couple of weeks, being careful to observe what happens. This is one mouthwash formulated from ingredients you would *want* absorbed into the oral tissues, including the sulcular wall. As mentioned earlier, you can be sensitive to one or more of the ingredients in any product, so no one product is appropriate for everyone. I have fourteen years combined experience observing the results of the two mouthwashes I recommend, and I have never seen any adverse reactions from either. Regardless, there still may be a few people out there who could be sensitive to something in one or the other product. On the other hand, I fail to grasp how it could possibly be considered a good idea to irrigate under the gum margins with any of the untouchables, but at least we all have a choice. With perhaps 90 percent of the public having some degree of gum disease right now, those wanting improvement would do well to choose their oral health products and devices more carefully.

You can go to the Hydrofloss website[10] for information and decide for yourself if this machine might benefit you. The information there concerning hydromagnetic technology pertains to the same technology found in the OxyCare 3000. All the supporting studies are there for you to download and review. Reading them will help you see how and why we can control what goes on in the sulcus. Having used an irrigator myself for a number of years, and having observed patients who use, or don't use, one themselves, I can tell you that it is invariably those using the irrigator who are the healthiest.

Once you enjoy the sensation of irrigation, you'll never go back to how your mouth feels when the microorganisms are winning. A mouth just isn't clean unless irrigation is done on a daily basis, and this oral health habit is a critical, often overlooked, factor in winning the oral health game. Until someone can see the bits and pieces of food debris, and get a whiff of the odors their irrigation efforts are flushing out from under their own gum margins, it is hard to imagine how contaminated that space we call the sulcus really is. Get yourself a hydromagnetic irrigator and apply what you have learned in this section; it is almost a certainty you will be glad you did.

WHY DON'T ALL DENTISTS RECOMMEND IRRIGATION?

One reason that irrigators are so infrequently recommended by dentists is because the dentists either don't recognize how critically important they are to oral health, or they believe that irrigation forces bacteria into the soft tissue, and consequently into the bloodstream. Irrigation does, in fact, have this effect, but it is temporary and can be ameliorated by the judicious use of antioxidants. Recent studies of CRP elevation in people with periodontal disease showed that just chewing gum elevated CRP 300 to 400 percent in these individuals because microorganisms pumped into the circulatory system cause inflammation, which is what triggers the CRP elevation. So, while irrigating the sulcus at a cleaning appointment every six months is beneficial, that's only one irrigation every 180 days or so. In order to be truly effective, sulcus cleansing has to be a daily part of cleaning the mouth.

Additionally, dentists differentiate between supragingival irrigation, which uses a tip that does not go into the sulcus, and subgingival irrigation, which uses very thin tips that can penetrate deeply into the sulcus. Either method can be effectively used in home care, especially when the patient is thoroughly instructed in the proper use of his or her new irrigator, and when either mouthwash I've recommended is used in the irrigant solution. Putting a mouthwash in your irrigant water that contains any of the nine ingredients that should never touch your lips, mouth, tongue, or sulcus (see Chapter 5) is not something I would ever recommend you do if you are serious about winning the oral health game.

8

Dr. Earl Mindell's Top Ten Nutrients for a Healthy Mouth

The most astonishing changes in my patients' oral health, energy levels, and attitudes has, by far, come from their taking advantage of my nutritional-supplement recommendations. All the oral health strategies discussed in this book are important, but in my opinion, appropriate nutritional supplementation for patients represents the wave of the future in health and wellness.

Any discussion of nutrition for oral health could easily double or triple the size of this book, but that would not serve our purposes here, as there are already quite a number of excellent books that have helped me develop the regimens I have formulated for patients, using Dr. Earl Mindell's products. For those of you who are really serious about health and wellness, a good place to start is with my coauthor's book *Earl Mindell's Vitamin Bible for the 21st Century.* With about 12 million copies of this book sold already, it's a classic, and its many pages cover a lot of very important information. From my perspective, as a dentist working with patients in the health and wellness arena, I have seen many of my patients experience profound improvements in oral and systemic health based solely on nutritional regimens aimed at oral health. My recommendations are *always* specific to oral health, since I practice dentistry, not medicine. However, the reality is that the mouth and its associated structures are connected to the rest of the body, and any nutritional supplements you take for dental reasons will obviously be disseminated throughout the entire body. I might want 100 percent of some nutritional supplement to go to inflamed gum tissues, for instance, but that's not the way our systems work. From a strictly dental perspective, however, I can make those nutritional-supplement recommendations for oral health, and the systemic health benefits that may also result become a welcome surprise for the patient. As more physicians and dentists turn to the use of nutritional supplements to help their patients, there will be a growing awareness of the multiple health benefits associated with certain supplements, such as the top ten nutritional supplements detailed in this chapter.

Before you can expect to benefit from the nutritional support associated with any particular supplement, it is critical for this supplement to be pure, have the actual amounts of ingredients in it that are stated on the label, and be highly absorbable in order to be bioavailable (capable of being used by the body). It would probably not surprise you to learn that there are vitamins (many of which you have probably seen recently in ads) that do not even dissolve on their way through the digestive system, and as reported in the *San Antonio Express-News* on March 8, 2003, the Food and Drug Administration has moved to impose new regulations upon dietary supplement manufacturers to force them to make clean, accurately labeled products. The article went on to say that the agency "is responding to many cases in which bacteria, glass, pesticides, lead, and other contaminants have been found in food supplements."[1] The agency was also responding to cases in which the supplements did not have the amounts of ingredients stated on the label; in fact, they usually had "much less" of the active ingredient than claimed. While this news probably doesn't shock and amaze anyone, it poses a problem for us if our patients go out and buy such products, and then expect to see results. Not only could they fail to get results, they could also run the risk of having additional problems from contaminated supplements. To the old saying about avoiding bargains on parachutes and brain surgery, we might add something about avoiding bargains on nutritional supplements.

With the wide range in quality as well as the cost and the considerable confusion about what's really necessary for optimal health, I recommend only pharmaceutical-grade supplements that use standardized extracts made from all-natural ingredients, all certified organic. This means that the supplement has the ingredients it says it has on the label, in the amounts stated, and is in a highly absorbable form, and that the supplement has ingredients that are certified free of chemical or biological residue. All-natural (plant) ingredients can be subjected to a wide array of contaminants, from pesticide residues to animal hair, and some of the products I recommend to patients have ingredients that come from as many as twenty-three countries, so even the sources of the ingredients must be carefully monitored. As a consumer, with literally hundreds of choices available, I can assure you I have done my due diligence, and while I wish the supplement industry would police itself, it hasn't yet, so you must do yours as well. Some very good products, besides the ones formulated by Dr. Mindell, are available, but for convenience, cost, quality, and bioavailability factors, as well as for consistent results and a no-risk money-back guarantee, his product line has my total confidence. My recommendations are on my website, and are based on the product line I use with my patients. (See "Contact Dr. Bonner" on page 122.)

I will endeavor to be precise in describing the dental health benefits associated with the top ten nutrients for a healthy mouth. Many of the known systemic health benefits of a specific nutrient will follow the dental benefits. Additionally, please note that all top ten nutrients listed are

THE TOP TEN NUTRIENTS IN ORDER OF IMPORTANCE

1. Vitamin C—Ascorbic Acid
2. Bioflavonoids—Citrus Bioflavonoids, Rutin, and Hesperidin (aka "Vitamin P")
3. Coenzyme Q_{10} (CoQ_{10})
4. Grapeseed Extract
5. Methylsulfonylmethane (MSM)
6. Vitamin E Complex and Selenium
7. Calcium and Magnesium
8. Green Tea Extract
9. Carotenoid Complex
10. B Complex

required for optimal health, but they are listed separately in order to describe their specific benefits to oral and systemic health. Someone could have optimal amounts of nine of the top ten nutrients and be deficient in CoQ_{10}, for example, and with a deficiency of CoQ_{10}, it is exceedingly unlikely that this person would be systemically or orally healthy. All the nutrients are important and all function synergistically, so leaving out any one of them will result in less than optimal health. Additionally, with some nutritional-supplement brands, or lines of products, getting all top ten in optimal amounts might be difficult or impossible, but with the line formulated by Dr. Mindell, taking the top ten daily can be as simple as taking just three products. I know for myself that if things aren't convenient and easy, consistent compliance is a problem for me, regardless of how important something may be. My patients have emphasized convenience as well, and taking the top ten is simplicity itself for most of them.

1. VITAMIN C—ASCORBIC ACID

Adequate circulating levels of vitamin C are required for healthy gum tissue and to prevent the deleterious effects of vitamin C deficiency. Most people associate this deficiency with sailors of days gone by whose swollen, bleeding gums, tooth loss, and sometimes death was caused by scurvy, the end result of a lack of vitamin C. But this deficiency did not go out of existence with the sailing ships; it's still here. Symptoms of scurvy still include bleeding and inflamed gums, as well as an impaired ability to heal. These exact conditions are seen more often than not in a large percentage of adult mouths, and it is my strong opinion that most people are vitamin C deficient.

Although vitamin C is relatively easy to obtain if you consume enough fruits and vegetables, most people don't, and they don't supplement with vitamin C either, and when those measures for good health aren't taken, a deficiency occurs. Additionally, the half-life for circulating vitamin C is just two to three hours, so maintaining optimal levels requires either taking several smaller doses throughout the day, or the use of timed-release formulations.

While the oral health benefits of vitamin C are presumably well-known, its appropriate use may also confer benefits that are well beyond discussing here. The *PDR for Nutritional Supplements* (First edition, 2001) has extensive information supporting that provided by Dr. Earl Mindell, and both these sources may compel the reader to reconsider the importance of vitamin C in the diet, and as a supplement. I feel most people would benefit from more vitamin C, more often, than is the norm at present.

One other very important use of vitamin C, based on its anti-inflammatory, antithrombotic, and vasodilatory activity, is its employment before periodontal procedures, including scaling and root planing or surgery.

Benefiting systemic health, vitamin C also:

- Decreases the severity and length of time for the common cold;
- Increases the effectiveness of prescription drugs to treat upper respiratory infections;
- Increases the absorption of inorganic iron;
- Decreases the effects of many allergy-producing substances;
- Decreases the incidence of blood clots in your veins;
- Decreases high blood pressure;
- Acts as an anticancer agent.

Dosage: 500–1,000 mg daily.

2. BIOFLAVONOIDS—CITRUS BIOFLAVONOIDS, RUTIN, AND HESPERIDIN (AKA "VITAMIN P")

Bioflavonoids, usually derived from lemons, oranges, and grapefruits, are required for the formation of collagen, the protein building block for gum tissue, cartilage, and bone. Bioflavonoids play an important role in maintaining a competent immune system. A Hungarian biochemist, Dr. Albert Szent-Györgyi, not only codiscovered ascorbic acid, or vitamin C, he also isolated a number of bioflavonoids and observed that the health of a coworker's gums improved more when flavonoids were combined with C, than when vitamin C was used alone. While Szent-Györgyi labeled flavonoids "vitamin P," bioflavonoids are not actually vitamins, so that designation has been dropped in favor of calling them flavonoids or bioflavonoids. These discoveries were made in the late 1920s, almost eighty years ago.

Since gum tissue is obviously on the front line as a barrier, and the formation of healthy gum tissue requires bioflavonoids, which are also required for a more competent immune system, optimal health requires a daily intake of bioflavonoids. Those who use BGSE Mint Toothpaste or BGSE Mint Mouthwash Treatment are applying bioflavonoids directly to oral soft tissues where they can be beneficially absorbed directly into inflamed tissues.

Bioflavonoids are especially important for further health-maintenance benefits, which are listed below. They are water-soluble nutrients, necessary for the proper functioning and absorption of vitamin C, and they also:

- Prevent vitamin C from being destroyed by free-radical oxygen molecules;
- Strengthen the tiny blood vessels on the surface of the skin, preventing bruising and black-and-blue marks;
- Build resistance to infection, and treat swelling and dizziness due to inner-ear disease.

Dosage: 500 mg daily.

3. COENZYME Q_{10} (CoQ_{10})

Coenzyme Q_{10} (CoQ_{10}) is so profoundly important to health that few adults should be doing without it as a nutritional supplement. CoQ_{10} is virtually *required* for the formation of collagen, which is a principal component of gum tissue and skin. Although CoQ_{10} is far better known for its heart-health and circulatory-system benefits, the *PDR for Nutritional Supplements* (First edition, 2001) states, "[CoQ_{10}] also appears to have usefulness in the management of periodontal disease in some," and additionally, "Significant CoQ_{10} deficiencies have been noted in diseased gingiva. CoQ_{10}'s efficacy in reducing gingival inflammation and periodontal pocket depth has been demonstrated in placebo-controlled trials" (pp. 103–104). In dental practice, the patient taking CoQ_{10} is not going to have an eye-popping experience right away with this supplement, since deficiencies can take weeks or months to resolve, but in time, many patients (and their dentist and hygienist) will note diminished bleeding, reduced or absent inflammation, and reduced pocket depth, including reattachment—and those are just some of the oral health observations.

There are some dosage guidelines for CoQ_{10} that must be observed for anyone to have any reasonable expectation of seeing results, or seeing any other health benefits from this supplement. The reason for these guidelines centers on the fact that CoQ_{10} is fat-soluble only, but the majority of the CoQ_{10} that people purchase is in a dry form. My chagrin over this situation is primarily because CoQ_{10} is, first of all, somewhat expensive; and second, the dry form most people take will only absorb about 25 percent of the CoQ_{10} amount stated on the label. If you take 50 mg of the dry form of CoQ_{10} twice daily expecting to get 100 mg of benefit, unless you have consumed CoQ_{10} with some amount of dietary fat, you would be fortunate to have absorbed even 25 mg—or just 25 percent of what you thought you were receiving. The form and amount of CoQ_{10} you need for optimal oral and systemic health couldn't be achieved in this example unless you took 400 mg a day. Like all supplements, but especially with the more expensive ones, being an informed consumer can make a very significant difference in money spent versus benefit received. There are some very good formulations of CoQ_{10} out there, including Dr. Mindell's product, so please don't cut corners on this supplement, and don't take the dry form. It is best to make sure you take optimal amounts of CoQ_{10} daily, but even suboptimal amounts are better than nothing.

CoQ_{10} has no known reactions with any prescription medications or drugs, and its safety has been clearly established, but its benefits in dentistry have not yet been even partially embraced by the profession. Medicine is way ahead of dentistry here, and CoQ_{10} is frequently recommended for its heart and circulatory system benefits, with healthier mouths being an occasionally observed bonus. It can work the other way around as well, and I eagerly anticipate that, with all the benefits that CoQ_{10} can safely provide for your health, its acceptance by dentistry (and medicine) will increase substantially in the future.

Supporting systemic health, Coenzyme Q_{10}:

- Reverses gum disease;
- Strengthens the heart muscle;
- Lowers high blood pressure.

Dosage: 60–180 mg daily.

4. GRAPESEED EXTRACT

Grapeseed and grape-skin extracts are antioxidant superstars called proanthocyanidins (PCOs) or oligomeric proanthocyanidins (OPC). PCO and OPC are used interchangeably. They offer oral and systemic health benefits, along with a total lack of toxicity, which make many health-oriented physicians and dentists recommend them almost universally.

Incorporating PCO extracts into a nutritional-supplement program offers total safety to the user as well as potential benefits orally and systemically that far outweigh any cost associated with this supplement. PCO extracts are exceedingly effective at inhibiting lipid peroxidation (inflammation) around atherosclerotic plaques, which is important because plaques that break free can block blood vessels, causing heart attacks, strokes, and so on.

PCOs have an extraordinary affinity for collagen. Blueberries are loaded with PCOs, so if you decide to grind up blueberries in the palms of your hands, be prepared for the PCO, in this case blue, to be attracted to the collagen in your skin, creating blue hands for a while.

The bottom line on PCO is to take the best all-natural standardized extract you can find, and take it twice daily.

Offering oral and systemic health benefits, PCOs:

- Support collagen structures and help prevent collagen degradation;
- Help create stronger collagen by helping to cross-link collagen fibers;
- Help prevent heart disease by protecting collagen, which is essential to healthy arteries;
- Help prevent free-radical damage;
- Inhibit enzymatic cleavage of collagen by enzymes;
- Help prevent the release of inflammation-inducing compounds;

- Strengthen small blood vessels;
- Act as powerful antioxidants.

Dosage: 100–200 mg daily.

5. METHYLSULFONYLMETHANE (MSM)

MSM is a totally nontoxic source of organic sulfur, and dental patients need this incredibly beneficial supplement for several reasons. One is that MSM can supply the organic sulfur for the sulfur-containing amino acids that are necessary for the formation of collagen. The sulcular wall is totally renewed every three to seven days, with the old cells being sloughed off into the sulcus; the new, healthy gum tissue requires lots of sulfur in order to be a more effective barrier. Most people are deficient in the dietary intake of sulfur, but because sulfur requirements in the diet have not yet been determined, you are on your own. Since MSM is also exceedingly anti-inflammatory, if you are taking it, you could expect a systematic reduction of inflammation, which could reduce joint pain due to arthritis or temporomandibular joint syndrome (TMJ), as well as relief from allergies and sinus problems (which can mimic tooth pain in upper teeth), and even relief from the pain associated with fibromyalgia. It is little wonder that most of the books on MSM have the word "miracle" somewhere in their title.

Once you know what MSM is about, you will begin to encounter people who could benefit from your knowledge. The alternatives people use have created a sad state of affairs: 50 to 80 percent of the people admitted to hospitals with gastrointestinal (GI) bleeding developed this condition through the use of what are termed NSAIDs (nonsteroidal anti-inflammatory drugs), the primary painkillers in use now. Every time someone is admitted with GI bleeding, they risk a 10 percent chance of dying.[2] At 76,000 hospitalizations a year, consuming NSAIDs for pain is a big problem. Remember MSM because many of the pain-causing problems people are taking NSAIDs for are treatable with MSM, which can be an extremely effective painkiller.

Besides being an anti-inflammatory, other dental benefits of MSM include its analgesic properties, its ability to dilate blood vessels and improve blood flow, and its ability to pass through cellular membranes, including the skin and gum tissue. MSM appears to be antimicrobial as well since it is known to kill parasites, including the protozoan *Giardia.*[3] If these benefits aren't enough by themselves, MSM also alters the cross-linking of collagen and can reduce scar tissue inside and outside the mouth.

Obviously, you should be taking MSM before surgical procedures are performed in order to expect any benefit. Also, because MSM can also cause loose stools in people new to taking it, they need to start at lower doses and work up to levels that offer the relief they are expecting. Crohn's disease, an inflammatory bowel condition, and ulcerative colitis can be positively affected by MSM, allowing anyone with these conditions to experience a decrease in symptoms and a more normal frequency and consistency in their bowel habits.[4]

To summarize, MSM is totally safe and its appropriate use by dental patients offers them a chance at healthier gum tissue, and faster healing with less discomfort and less scarring. MSM powder, in combination with antioxidants and absorption-enhancing ingredients, such as vitamin C, makes an exceptional toothbrushing powder, and if you swallow the mix, you get many systemic benefits as well. Use one-half teaspoon of MSM (about 2 grams). The mouth needs to be rinsed after brushing, since vitamin C is ascorbic acid, and it can and will dissolve enamel if left in contact with the teeth. (Although the manufacturer of the MSM powder I recommend doesn't suggest this particular regimen for the product, daily midday use over the last three years has not hurt my teeth at all.)

MSM needs to be a part of virtually every adult's daily regimen, and the best dosage really depends upon the individual need. As one of the top ten nutrients for oral health, I hope you find MSM to be of benefit.

This organic sulfur compound, found in plant and animal tissues, comes in a variety of forms, including tablets, capsules, and powder, as well as lotions for topical use. As a systemic health promoter, MSM:

- Reduces allergic symptoms;
- Relieves pain and inflammation due to arthritis;
- Promotes wound healing.

Dosage: 1,000–9,000 mg daily, in divided doses.

6. VITAMIN E COMPLEX AND SELENIUM

Vitamin E is a potent antioxidant that is necessary to help gum tissue heal. While vitamin E is better known for its cardioprotective effects, especially its ability to prevent the oxidation of LDL cholesterol (a step in the development of atherosclerosis), vitamin E's role in maintaining healthy gum tissue is most likely due to its ability to facilitate the immune system. Remember, the sulcular soft tissue wall is in intimate contact with a potentially very toxic chemical and microbiological stew that is capable of initiating an immune response, which creates inflammation and a cascade of events that can have very serious consequences. Only the natural, or d- forms of vitamin E complex should be used, as synthetic l- forms cannot be used by the body. Additionally, l-forms can interfere with the natural d- forms and prevent optimal utilization of the forms the body is capable of using.

Natural vitamin E can be applied directly to sore, inflamed gum tissue, up to three times daily, as a soothing, healing measure. Of course, professional dental care should be sought for a definitive diagnosis and possible treatment.

Selenium is an exceedingly potent antioxidant that tunes up the immune system. This potent antioxidant needs to be incorporated in a supplement regimen to improve the gum tissue's ability to resist chemical, enzymatic, gaseous, and microbiological insults, all of which can occur in the sulcus.

There are eight tocopherols: alpha, beta, delta, epsilon, eta, gamma, theta, and zeta as well as the interrelated tocotrienols and selenium, all of which when combined offer synergistic antioxidant protection.

Vitamin E (tocopherol):

- Slows the aging process;
- Prevents oxidation of bad cholesterol;
- Supplies oxygen to the body to give more endurance;
- Protects the lungs against air pollution;
- Prevents and dissolves blood clots;
- Alleviates fatigue;

- Decreases the risk of heart disease and strokes.

Dosage: 400–800 IU daily.

Tocotrienols—The Vitamin E Complex for the 21st Century:

- Decreases serum cholesterol, while fighting bad cholesterol and promoting good cholesterol;
- Fights hardening of the arteries, which can lead to heart attacks and stroke.

Dosage: 400–800 IU daily.

Selenium (usually taken with vitamin E):

- Decreases the risk of developing cancer, heart disease, and strokes;
- Is an antioxidant.

Dosage: 100–200 mcg daily.

7. CALCIUM AND MAGNESIUM

It is probably news to no one that adequate amounts of calcium and magnesium are required for healthy bone growth and maintenance. Advertising has done its job. However, what may be news is that many of the calcium supplements people purchase and consume fail to dissolve, thus rendering their bioavailability to just about zero. In other words, these supplements are a waste of money, and even worse, they offer no health benefit. With the incidence of osteoporosis increasing, especially in the United States, it is becoming more important than ever both to take supplements that work and to decrease the consumption of substances known to deplete calcium (soft drinks, for instance). In addition to the role of calcium and magnesium in maintaining bone health, a healthy mouth requires these nutrients for nerve and muscle function. Magnesium is also needed for energy production. Dietary sources alone do not provide adequate levels of either nutrient, so you should consider supplementing with both. The product I recommend (and take) is formulated for maximum bioavailability (it totally disintegrates in less than one minute when placed in plain water).

Calcium and magnesium are nature's tranquilizers. They:

- Maintain strong bones and healthy teeth;
- Decrease the risk of bone loss and fractures;
- Decrease the risk of colon cancer;
- Keep your heart beating regularly;
- Alleviate insomnia;
- Help maintain normal weight;
- Help burn fat and produce energy;
- Fight depression;
- Help prevent heart attacks;
- Help prevent calcium deposits, kidney stones, and gallstones;
- Alleviate premenstrual syndrome (PMS).

*Dosage: Calcium 1,000–1,*200 mg daily. Magnesium 500–600 mg daily.

8. GREEN TEA EXTRACT

Green tea and green tea extracts offer numerous oral and systemic health benefits. For starters, the current dental literature is recognizing that green tea can literally reverse a significant percentage of oral cancers. While I am recommending green tea as a preventive, since oral cancer should obviously be treated by a medical or dental professional, green tea has substances in it that tell abnormal cells to undergo cell suicide, or apoptosis. How this mechanism works is unclear, but suffice it to say that the majority of my patients are directed to drink at least three cups of tea daily by swishing the liquid around in their mouths before swallowing it.

There are many benefits to my patients, but I am primarily interested in the anti-cavity, antibacterial, antiviral benefits, as well as the anticancer and antithrombotic (preventing dangerous blood clots) benefits associated with drinking green tea. In the mouth, green tea helps destroy the biofilm, creating cleaner teeth and oral soft tissues. One study demonstrated that it can reduce dental decay by inhibiting the growth of *Streptococcus mutans*,[5] while another study showed that the green tea catechins (crystalline substances) actually destroyed *Streptococcus mutans*.[6]

If you are on blood thinners, green tea can enhance their effect, so consult with your physician before drinking green tea. Otherwise, find a green tea you like and make it a habit to consume several cups a day. Considering that the Japanese consume very large quantities of green tea and they also have the longest life spans of any nationality in the world, I strongly encourage you to take advantage of this powerful nutrient.

Providing myriad health benefits, green tea:

- Is rich in polyphenols, which are powerful antioxidants;
- Inhibits the formation of cancerous tumors;
- Can heal sun-damaged skin;
- Has strong anticancer properties.

Dosage: 100–200 mg daily.

9. CAROTENOID COMPLEX

Some members of the carotenoid complex, especially alpha-carotene and beta-carotene, are essential for oral health, since the body can convert either substance into vitamin A as needed. Vitamin A is necessary for the maintenance of mucous membranes (which make up most of the inside of the mouth—cheeks, lips, under the tongue, the posterior aspect of the roof of the mouth and throat, and all the gum tissue except for the part attached to the bone and directly around the teeth). With this in mind, it is not a good idea to be deficient in either of these carotenoids. The additional three carotenoids listed in this section (lutein, lycopene, and zeaxanthin) offer powerful benefits to oral soft tissues as well, but are becoming much better known for their ability to retard or prevent the diseases mentioned below. Consume lots of the brightly colored fruits and vegetables, and make sure you take an optimal amount of a carotenoid supplement as insurance.

Carotenoids are powerful natural chemicals that act as antioxidants and have anticancer properties. Fifty carotenoids are found in edible orange, yellow, red, and green fruits and vegetables. Following are the five most important carotenoids.

Alpha-Carotene:

- Converts to vitamin A if needed by the body;
- Decreases tumors in animals;
- Is ten times more powerful than beta-carotene in protecting skin, eyes, liver, and lung tissue from free-radical damage.

Dosage: In a complex with beta-carotene, 10,000–20,000 IU daily.

Beta-Carotene:

- Converts to vitamin A if needed by the body;
- Strengthens the immune system;
- Decreases the risk of hardening of the arteries;
- Decreases the risk of heart disease and strokes;
- Protects against cataract formation.

Dosage: In a complex with alpha-carotene, 10,000–20,000 IU daily.

Lutein:

- Protects the eyes and retards macular degeneration.

Dosage: 6–20 mg daily.

Lycopene:

- Inhibits the growth of cancer cells;

- Decreases the risk of prostate cancer;
- Protects against tobacco smoke and exposure to UV rays of the sun.

Dosage: 6–10 mg daily.

Zeaxanthin:

- Protects the eyes;
- Retards macular degeneration of the retina;
- Has anticancer properties.

Dosage: 30–130 mg daily.

10. B COMPLEX

This group comprises the largest number of water-soluble nutrients. Vitamin B complex can include B_1 (thiamine), B_2 (riboflavin), B_3 (niacin), B_5 (pantothenic acid), B_6 (pyridoxine HCL), B_{12} (cyanocobalamin), and folate (another member of the B group sometimes known as vitamin M).

Vitamins B_2, B_3, B_6, and B_{12} are all closely associated with promoting oral health. Deficiencies in these vitamins are associated with sore, inflamed oral mucosal tissues (sometimes fiery red and very inflamed) as well as cracking at the corners of the mouth. B complex is intimately associated with the production of energy and energy release and is involved in amino-acid metabolism (amino acids combine to make proteins—and gum tissue, mucosa, and skin are mostly protein), so without B complex in optimal amounts, a healthy mouth and any other mucosal or skin structures are likely unachievable. Many cereals contain some of the B-complex vitamins as additives, but while this may help some achieve RDA levels of this important complex on an occasional basis, the RDA is so far below the levels required for optimal health that it is considered a joke in the alternative health world. The RDA refers only to the levels required to avoid serious disease.

Additionally, B complex is important for:

- Energy production;
- Relieving postoperative dental pain;

- Treating herpes zoster (shingles);
- Improving mental attitude;
- Aiding in digestion, especially carbohydrates;
- Promoting healthy skin, hair, and nails;
- Helping to eliminate sore mouth, lips, and tongue;
- Benefiting vision and alleviating eye fatigue;
- Reducing cholesterol and triglycerides.

B complex also:

- Decreases the severity of migraine headaches;
- Enhances circulation and lowers high blood pressure;
- Treats vertigo;
- Helps eliminate bad breath;
- Lowers the risk of heart disease;
- Strengthens the immune system;
- Prevents kidney stone formation;
- Alleviates nausea, including morning sickness;
- Helps reduce dry mouth caused by antidepressants;
- Decreases muscle spasms, leg cramps, and hand numbness;
- Forms and regenerates red blood cells, preventing anemia;
- Promotes growth and appetite in children;
- Relieves irritability;
- Improves concentration, memory, and balance;
- Helps keep hair from turning gray;
- Protects against neurotubular defect of the newborn;
- Improves lactation;

- Aids liver function;
- Protects against intestinal parasites and food poisoning;
- Acts as a pain reliever;
- Aids in wound healing;
- Builds antibodies to fight infection;
- Treats postoperative shock;
- Prevents fatigue;
- Reduces adverse and toxic effects of many antibiotics.

Dosage: 50–100 mg daily.

Conclusion

As I mentioned early in this book, someone once stated, "If you keep doing what you've been doing, you'll keep getting what you've been getting," and by now you know that gum disease is potentially a very serious systemic disease. This book is about change, and while few people like change for any reason, neither you, as a person concerned about your health, nor I, as a responsible dentist, can sit back and do the same old things and expect different results.

I'm cautiously optimistic that many of you have discovered something in these pages that will help you decide to do something different, and that, by implementing changes—even something as simple as using a safe and effective toothpaste—you'll experience noticeable health benefits that will reward you for taking a proactive and informed role in your general health and wellness. The pursuit of these states is a journey, not a destination, and the more information you have, the better you'll be able to decide for yourself what's right for you. I hope this book will be helpful in your journey toward health.

A Note from the Luckiest Person on Earth—Bill Barfield

By all rights, I should already be back with my maker (several times), but because of much good luck, I am here still and writing these words. Meeting Dr. Michael Bonner, and his refusal to clean my teeth, is a big part of my continued good fortune. Dr. Bonner's dedication to the improvement of health and the quality of life through nutrition has not only improved my gum condition, but I am certain it spared me from having another angioplasty procedure, or worse yet, coronary bypass surgery.

Let me give you a little history about my health condition. At the age of twenty-eight, I had my first angioplasty because the left anterior descending artery was 97 percent blocked. In the several decades since, I have undergone fourteen angioplasties and had five stents placed in the various arteries connected to the heart. All this is mainly due to genetics, as my cholesterol and blood pressure are normal, and my weight is only slightly above recommended levels, the only negative factor being that I have smoked since the age of twelve. I am lucky to be alive in a time when the medical profession is capable of performing angioplasty. My mother was not so fortunate because she died from hardening of her arteries at age forty-one. I am also lucky in that I can tell to within 4 to 5 percent how much blockage I have in the arteries, once I hit 50 to 60 percent blockage.

In terms of dentistry, prior to moving to San Antonio where I met Dr. Bonner, I had undergone two previous periodontal treatments in St. Louis and was on a quarterly cleaning procedure. My first dentist in San

Antonio would only clean my teeth every six months, and was more interested in performing cosmetic procedures than in preventing the return of gum disease. I got lucky again when my employer switched our dental insurance carrier, forcing me to find another dentist, who turned out to be Dr. Bonner.

I take two prescription medications (Toprol and Zocor) and a daily aspirin for my heart condition. Over time, I had haphazardly added vitamin and mineral supplements to my daily regimen (vitamins B, C, E, calcium, and selenium) after reading or hearing about the benefits of their use. Even on this regimen, however, I had six to eight of my angioplasties and received all five stents.

When I met Dr. Bonner, all I wanted him to do was clean my teeth. After looking at my mouth, he started talking about nutritional health improvement, systemic this and that, and something called coenzyme Q_{10}. When he asked me how I was feeling, I told him I thought one of my rear teeth was hurting and could be decayed. "Oh yes," he replied, "you have gum disease again, that is why your teeth are hurting." Then, with a little camera, he went around my mouth, showing me some bleeding around two different teeth when he just poked them with his fingers. And he wiggled one of them to demonstrate how extremely loose it was. He then asked if I knew there was a link between gum disease and heart problems, and repeated his question about how I was feeling.

This was kind of shocking to me because I felt I was about 75 or 80 percent blocked, but had not yet said anything, even to my wife. Still, he knew, so I admitted that I would probably have to have another angioplasty in about a month, but I just wanted him to clean my teeth.

Dr. Bonner then told me that there were a number of cases where a person with periodontal disease would have a tooth cleaning and then would have a heart attack. He stated flat out that he would not clean my teeth until my general health had improved, and then suggested that I read a couple of books, visit a website on periodontal nutrition, and discuss my condition and any changes I might need to make with my cardiologist and primary-care physician. Needless to say, I left his office frustrated, thinking I would have to find another dentist who accepted this new employer's dental insurance just so I could get someone to clean my teeth.

My luck continued, though, when I decided I would visit Dr. Bonner's website on my new, faster computer. (I'm sure if I still had my old PC, I would not have done so, and might still be looking for another dentist.) When I read about the link between gum disease and cardiac problems on the website, it was like I was reading my own medical history. As I got deeper into the site, I discovered that it led to the sale of nutritional supplements produced by FreeLife. This made me very skeptical and, in fact, I so stated to Dr. Bonner when he called me the next day to see how I was feeling and answer any questions I might have.

His response to my questioning attitude was truthful and insightful. He simply said that studies show, if you can give people access to recommended information, products, services, and so on, they are more likely to take advantage of this information than if you leave them on their own to find it. As I thought about that, I realized that my cardiologist had his own stress test and cardiac catheterization lab, and my primary-care physician had his own x-ray and blood-work facilities. Just like them, Dr. Bonner has his own outlet, which would save me from having to run to various stores to find any nutritional products he recommended. Besides, their quality is monitored by the doctors who produce them, and by the doctors, like Dr. Bonner, who see the benefits of them.

Having resolved that in my mind, I printed out much of the material on the FreeLife products and discovered that they contained everything I was already taking or thinking about taking, plus other ingredients such as coenzyme Q_{10}. I then read the books Dr. Bonner recommended, and my wife and I discussed the entire situation, including finding another dentist.

Despite all our reservations and skepticisms, my wife and I decided to continue with Dr. Bonner and to try the program he recommended (Basic Mindell Plus and Cardio Mate). We added Zincosamine for the joints and started using BGSE toothpaste, which amazingly makes our teeth noticeably cleaner.

Within one month, my gum infection had cleared up, the gum swelling had receded, a healthy pink color had returned to my gums, and my loose tooth had become tighter. When Dr. Bonner probed my gums in several areas, he could find absolutely no bleeding or probing depths beyond a few millimeters, which was not the case before I started the nutrition and oral health program. But more important to me,

I no longer feel that my arteries are as blocked as they were when I started the program. I am certain that if I were to have a cardiac cath performed today, my arteries would be less than 50 percent blocked. I have become a firm believer in the benefits of nutritional health and the use of the products that Dr. Bonner recommended, and I have every expectation of being a long-term patient and student of his.

Thank you, Dr. Bonner, for your contagious and almost monomaniacal commitment to nutritional health. You have opened my eyes to new possibilities, which are leading me to a much brighter future. Now, can you clean my teeth? And, by the way, can you also tell me how to easily kick this smoking habit?

Sincerely,
Bill Barfield
San Antonio, Texas

References

Allen, J. E. "Chronic infections can lead to heart disease." *San Antonio Express-News* (26 March 2001).

Altman, R. D., and K. C. Marcussen. "Effects of a ginger extract on knee pain in patients with osteoarthritis." *Arthritis and Rheumatism* 44 (11) (2001): 2531–2538.

Balch, James. *The Super Antioxidants: Why They Will Change the Face of Healthcare in the 21st Century.* New York, NY: M. Evans and Company, Inc., 1998.

Balch, James, and Phyllis Balch. *Prescription for Nutritional Healing,* Third Edition. New York, NY: Avery/Penguin Putnam Inc., 2000.

Barney, Paul. *Doctor's Guide to Natural Medicine.* Orem, UT: Woodland Publishing, Inc., 1998.

Beck, J. D. "Epidemiology of periodontal disease in older adults." In *Periodontal Care for Older Adults,* ed. R. P. Ellen, 9–35. Toronto, Canada: Canadian Scholars Press Inc., 1991.

Beck, J. D., R. I. Garcia, G. Heiss, et al. "Periodontal disease and cardiovascular disease." *Journal of Periodontal Care* 67 (1996):1123–1137.

Beck, J. D., S. Offenbacher, R. Williams, et al. "Periodontitis: a risk factor for coronary heart disease?" *Annals of Periodontology* 3 (1998):127–141.

Bland, J. *Vitamin C: The Future Is Now.* New Canaan, CT: Keats Publishing, 1995.

Bliznakov, E. G., and G.L. Hunt. *The Miracle Nutrient: Coenzyme Q_{10}.* New York, NY: Bantam, 1987.

Chadda, S., R. Dunford, R. Genco, et al. "Periodontal disease is a predictor of cardiovascular disease in a Native American population." *Journal of Dental Res* 76 (1997):48.

Cheraskin, E. *Vitamin C: Who Needs It?* Birmingham, AL: Arlington Press, 1993.

Destefano, F., R. F. Anda, H. S. Kahn, et al. "Dental disease and risk of coronary heart disease and mortality." *British Medical Journal* 306 (1993): 688–691.

Dragsholt, M. T. "A new causal model of dental diseases associated with endocarditis." *Annals of Periodontology* 3 (1998):184–196.

Frei, B., L. England, and B. N. Ames. "Ascorbate is an outstanding antioxidant in human blood plasma." *Proceedings of the National Academy of Science* 86 (1989):6377–6381.

Ginter, E. "Optimum intake of vitamin C for the human organism." *Nutr Health* 1 (1982):66–77.

Grau, A. J., F. Buggle, C. Ziegler, et al. "Association between acute cerebrovascular ischemia and chronic and recurrent infection." *Stroke* 28 (1997):1724–1729.

Hanioka, T., et al. "Therapy with coenzyme Q_{10} for patients with periodontal disease. Effect of coenzyme Q_{10} on the immune system." *Journal of Dental Health* 43 (1993):667–672.

Havsteen, B. "Flavonoids, a class of natural products of high pharmacological potency." *Biochemical Pharmacology* 32 (1983):1141–1148.

Hertog, M. G., et al. "Dietary antioxidant flavonoids and risk of coronary heart disease: The Zutphen Elderly Study." *The Lancet* 342 (1993): 1007–1011.

Herzberg, M. C., and M. W. Meyer. "Dental plaque, platelets and cardiovascular diseases." *Annals of Periodontology* 3 (1998):151–160.

Hobbs, C., and E. Haas. *Vitamins for Dummies.* Foster City, CA: IDG Books Worldwide, Inc., 1999.

Iwamoto, Y., et al. "Clinical effects of coenzyme Q_{10} on periodontal disease." *Biomedical and Clinical Aspects of Coenzyme Q_{10}* 3 (1981): 109–119.

Jacob, S., R. Lawrence, and M. Zucker. *The Miracle of MSM: The Natural Solution for Pain.* New York, NY: Berkley Books, 1999.

Jamieson, J., L. E. Dorman, and V. Marriott. *Growth Hormone: Reversing Human Aging Naturally.* New Canaan, CT: Safe Goods, 1997.

Joshipura, K., C. Douglass, and W. C. Willett. "Possible explanations for the tooth loss and cardiovascular disease relationship." *Annals of Periodontology* 3 (1998): 175–183.

Kinane, D. F. "Periodontal disease's contributions to cardiovascular disease: an overview of potential mechanisms." *Annals of Periodontology* 3 (1998): 142–150.

Kiuchi, F., et al. "Inhibition of prostaglandin and leukotriene biosynthesis by gingerols and diaryheptanoids." *Chemical Pharmacology Bulletin* 40 (1992): 387–391.

Kiuchi, F., M. Shibuyu, and U. Sankawa. "Inhibitors of prostaglandin biosynthesis from ginger." *Chemical Pharmacology Bulletin* 30 (1982):754–757.

Klatz, R. *New Anti-Aging Secrets for Maximum Lifespan.* Chicago, IL: Sports Tech Labs, Inc. 1999.

Klatz, R., and R. Goldman. *7 Anti-Aging Secrets for Optimal Digestion and Scientific Weight Loss.* Chicago, IL: Elite Sports Medicine Publications, 1996.

———*Stopping the Clock.* New Canaan, CT: Keats Publishing, Inc., 1996.

Lee, W. *Coenzyme Q_{10}: Is It Our New Fountain of Youth?* New Canaan, CT: Keats Publishing, Inc., 1987.

Loesche, W. J., A. Schork, M. S. Terpenning, et al. "The relationship between dental disease and cerebral vascular accident in elderly United States veterans." *Annals of Periodontology* 3 (1998):161–174.

Loew, G. D. "Etiopathogenesis of cardiovascular disease: hemostasis, thrombosis and vascular medicine." *Annals of Periodontology* 3 (1998):121–126.

Majeed, M., V. Badmaev, U. Shivakumar, et al. *Curcuminoids: Antioxidant Phytonutrients.* Piscataway, NJ: NutriScience Publishers, Inc. 1995.

Matilla, K. J. "Dental infections and coronary atherosclerosis." *Atherosclerosis* 103 (1993):205–211.

Matilla, K. J, M. S. Nieminen, V. V. Valtonen, et al. "Association between dental health and acute myocardial infarction." *British Medical Journal* 298 (1989): 779–782.

McRee, J. T., et al. "Therapy with coenzyme Q_{10} for patients with periodontal disease. Effect of coenzyme Q_{10} on subgingival microorganisms." *Journal of Dental Health* 43 (1993):659–666.

Mindell, E. *Earl Mindell's Vitamin Bible for the 21st Century.* New York, NY: Warner Books, Inc., 1999.

———.*The MSM Miracle: Enhance Your Health with Organic Sulfur.* New Canaan, CT: Keats Publishing, Inc., 1997.

Mindell, E., and V. Hopkins. *Dr. Earl Mindell's What You Should Know About the Super Antioxidant Miracle.* New Canaan, CT: Keats Publishing, Inc., 1996.

———.*Dr. Earl Mindell's What You Should Know About Natural Health for Men.* New Canaan, CT: Keats Publishing, Inc., 1996.

———.*Dr. Earl L. Mindell's What You Should Know About Nutrition for Active Lifestyles.* New Canaan, CT: Keats Publishing, Inc., 1996.

Murray, M. T. *Encyclopedia of Nutritional Supplements.* Rocklin, CA: Prima Publishing, 1996.

Nery, E. D., F. Meister, R. F. Ellinger, et al. "Prevalence of medical problems in periodontal patients obtained from three different populations." *Journal of Clinical Periodontalogy* 58 (1987):564–568.

Page, R. C. "The pathobiology of periodontal diseases may affect systemic diseases: inversion of a paradigm." *Annals of Periodontology* (1998): 108–120.

PDR for Nutritional Supplements. 1st ed. Montvale, NJ: Medical Economics Company, Inc., 2001.

Sachs, Allan. *Grapefruit Seed Extract.* Mendocino, CA: LifeRhythm, 1997.

Shabert, J., and N. Ehrlich. *The Ultimate Nutrient: Glutamine.* Garden City Park, NY: Avery Publishing Group, 1994.

Simon, J. A. "Vitamin C and cardiovascular disease: a review." *Journal of the American College of Nutrition* 11 (1992):107–125.

Sinatra, S. *L-Carnitine and the Heart.* New Canaan, CT: Keats Publishing, Inc., 1999.

———. *The Coenzyme Q_{10} Phenomenon.* Chicago, IL: Keats, Div. of NTC/ Contemporary Publishing Group, Inc., 1998.

Sinatra, S., J. Sinatra, and R. J. Lieberman. *Heart Sense for Women, Your Plan for Natural Prevention and Treatment.* Washington, DC: LifeLine Press, 2000.

Taylor, N. *Green Tea: The Natural Secret for a Healthier Life.* New York, NY: Kensington Publishing Company, 1998.

Tixier, J. M, et al. "Evidence by in vivo and in vitro studies that binding of pycnogenols to elastin affects its rate of degradation by elastases." *Biochemical Pharmacology* 33 (1984):3933–3939.

Udall, K. G. *Flaxseed Oil: The Premier Source of Omega-3 Fatty Acids.* Orem, UT: Woodland Publishing, 1998.

Wehrmacher, W. H. "Periodontal disease predicts and possibly contributes to acute myocardial infarction." *Dentistry Today* (April 2001):80–81.

Wilkenson, E. G., R. M. Arnold, and K. Folkers. "Treatment of periodontal and other soft tissue diseases of the oral cavity with coenzyme Q_{10}." In *Biomedical and Clinical Aspects of Coenzyme Q_{10}* 1 (1977):251–265.

Endnotes

Chapter 1

1. Tonzentich, J., "Sources, measurements and implications of oral malodor: abstract," *International Academy of Dental Research (IADR) Symposium,* Acapulco, Mexico, April 1991.

2. *San Antonio Express-News,* April 8, 2003, Section D, Page 1.

3. "High CRP Bodes Ill for Heart Health," *San Antonio Express-News,* May 5, 2003, Section C, pages 1 and 3.

Chapter 2

1. Balch, James, and Phyllis Balch. *Prescription for Nutritional Healing,* Third Edition, New York, NY, Avery Div. Penguin Putnam, 2000, p. 564.

2. AAP website: http://www.perio.org/consumer/mediahg1.html. From online article, "Healthier Gums, Healthier Bodies!" Chicago, July 9, 1998.

3. http://www.seratec.com/seiten/cr220.html

4. "High CRP Bodes Ill for Heart Health," *San Antonio Express-News,* May 5, 2003, Section C, pages 1 and 3.

5. Noack, B., Genco, R. J., Trevisan, M., et al., "Periodontal infections contribute to elevated systemic C-reactive protein level," *Journal of Periodontology,* September 2001; pages 1221–1227.

Chapter 3

1. Klatz, Ronald M., *New Anti-Aging Secrets for Maximum Lifespan,* Chicago, IL, Sports Tech Labs, Inc., 1999, page 53.

2. Geerts, S.O., Nys, M., De Mol, P., et al., "Systemic release of endotoxins induced by gentle mastication: association with periodontitis severity," *Journal of Periodontology,* January 2002: 73–77.

Chapter 4

1. Farr, Cheryl, "The best advances in dentistry in the past 15 years," *Dentistry Today,* February 18, 2000; 2:62.

2. The *PDR for Nutritional Supplements* is a good resource and is available at larger bookstores or at 1-800-678-5689.

3. Gomolka, K., "Perio/Systemic Conference: special report: periodontal disease and cardiac conditions: association or coincidence?" *Dental Products Report,* December 2001: 46–81. ADA symposium's first installment in a series titled, "Taking Oral Health to Heart."

4. *Dentistry Today,* December 2001; 14: 80.

5. Gomolka, K., "Perio/Systemic Conference: special report: periodontal disease and cardiac conditions: association or coincidence?" *Dental Products Report,* December 2001:46–81. ADA symposium's first installment in a series titled, "Taking Oral Health to Heart."

6. "Perio Disease and Cardiac Conditions: Association or Coincidence?" *Dental Products Report,* December 2001: 48–49.

7. "Perio Disease and Cardiac Conditions: Association or Coincidence?" *Dental Products Report,* December 2001: 50.

8. Zincosamine was the subject of a large study published December 2001, in the *Journal of Arthritis and Rheumatology.*

Chapter 5

1. The web address for Linda Chaé is www.lindachae.com.

Chapter 6

1. Tonzentich, J., "Sources, measurements and implications of oral malodor: abstract," International Academy of Dental Research (IADR) Symposium. Acapulco, Mexico. April 1991.

2. Ford, Earl S., "Body mass index, diabetes, and C-reactive protein among U.S. adults," *Diabetes Care,* December 1999.

3. Ridker, P.M., Cushman, M., Stampfer, M.J., et al., "Inflammation, aspirin and the risk of cardiovascular disease in apparently healthy men," *New England Journal of Medicine,* 1997; 336: 973–979.

4. Gregg, Robert H, McCarthy, Delwin K., Co-Directors, Institute for Advanced Laser Dentistry: Letters from Readers, page 22 of a letter covering parts of pages 18, 20, 22, and 90, *Dental Economics,* August 2002.

5. National Institutes of Health will give you access to the health information you want. Available at http://health.nih.gov.

Chapter 7

1. Hattori, M., Kusumoto, I.T., Namba, T., et al., "Effect of tea polyphenols on glucan synthesis by glucotrasferase from Streptococcus mutans," *Chemical Pharmacology Bulletin,* 1990; 38 (3): 717–720.

2. Taylor, Nadine, Green Tea. New York, NY: Kensington Publishing Corp., 1998, p. 73. The study quoted is Sakanaka S., Kim, M., Taniguchi, M., et al., "Antibacterial substances in Japanese green tea extract against Streptococcus mutans, a cariogenic bacterium," *Agric. Biol. Chem.*, 1989; 53 (9): 2307–2311.

3. Ibid.

4. Hikino, H., Kiso, Y., Hatano, T., et al., "Antihepatotoxic actions of tannins," *Journal of Ethnopharmacology,* 1985; 14:19.

5. Kutten, N.A.A., Narayana, N., Moghadam, B.K.H., "Desquamative stomatitis associated with the routine use of oral health care products," *General Dentistry,* November–December 2001: 596–602.

6. Watt, D.L., Rosenfelder, C., Sutton, C.D., "The effect of oral irrigation with a magnetic water treatment device on plaque and calculus," *Journal of Clinical Periodontology,* May 1993: 314–317.

7. *Journal of Clinical Periodontology,* May 1998: 316–321.

8. "Diet, nutrition, and oral health: a rational approach for the dental practice," *Journal of the American Dental Association,* 1984; 109: 20–32.

9. Genco, R.J., "Current view of risk factors for periodontal diseases," *Journal of Periodontal,* 1996; 67: 1041–1049.

10. The website for Hydrofloss is www.hydrofloss.com. The phone number is 1-800-635-3594.

Chapter 8

1. *San Antonio Express-News,* April 8, 2003, Section D, Page 1.

2. Jacob, S.W., Lawrence, R.M., Zucker, M., *The Miracle of MSM: The Natural Solution for Pain,* New York, NY: Berkley Books, 1999, p. 73.

3. Ibid, p. 23.

4. Ibid, p. 77.

5. Hattori, M., Kusumoto, I.T., Namba, T., et al., "Effect of tea polyphenols on glucan synthesis by glucotrasferase from Streptococcus mutans," *Chemical Pharmacology Bulletin,* 1990; 38 (3): 717–720.

6. Sakanaka, S., Kim, M., Taniguchi, M., et al., "Antibacterial substances in Japanese green tea extract against Streptococcus mutans, a cariogenic bacterium," *Agricultural Biological Chemistry,* 1989; 53 (9): 2307–2311.

Contact Dr. Bonner

Michael P. Bonner, D.D.S.
P.O. Box 1347
Rockdale, TX 76567

www.oralhealthbible.com
dr@oralhealthbible.com

1-877-815-4933 (voicemail)
1-210-699-0103 (fax)

Index

About the Authors

Dr. Michael P. Bonner practices dentistry full time in Rockdale, Texas, with another dentist, three dental hygienists, and six very busy staff members. He has also found time to lecture on dental health and wellness topics to physicians and dentists nationwide and abroad, including Aruba, Canada, Malaysia, and Singapore. Dr. Bonner has authored numerous articles in newspapers, newsletters, and magazines on topics related to health and wellness.

Dr. Bonner majored in chemistry and biology at East Texas State University (now Texas A&M at Commerce) and graduated with a Bachelor of Science degree in 1969. He attended dental school at the University of Texas Health Science Center, San Antonio, receiving his D.D.S. degree in 1975.

He is a member of several professional organizations including the Academy of General Dentistry, the American Academy of Anti-Aging Medicine, the American Dental Association, the Texas Dental Association, and the San Antonio District Dental Society.

Dr. Bonner has been an active flight instructor for thirty-six years, and also travels about 25,000 miles annually on either of his two BMW motorcycles. A Civil War enthusiast, he tours the battlefields and collects history books on the subject.

Dr. Earl L. Mindell is a founder of the health and wellness revolution and the author of more than thirty books, including *The Vitamin Bible,* which has sold more than 10 million copies worldwide. A registered pharmacist, a master herbalist, and an internationally recognized expert on nutrition, drugs, vitamins, and herbal remedies, Dr. Mindell is a Professor of Nutrition at Pacific Western University in Los Angeles. He lives in Beverly Hills, California.

www.ingramcontent.com/pod-product-compliance
Lightning Source LLC
Chambersburg PA
CBHW050220270326
41914CB00003BA/506

* 9 7 8 1 6 8 1 6 2 8 1 4 1 *